Pharmacological

CLASSIFICATION OF DRUGS

with Doses and Preparations

Pharmacological
CLASSIFICATION OF DRUGS
with Doses and Preparations

SEVENTH EDITION

KD Tripathi MD
Formerly-Director-Professor and Head of Pharmacology
Maulana Azad Medical College and associated
LNJP and GB Pant Hospitals, New Delhi

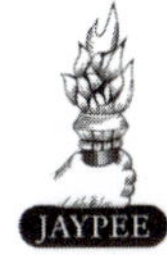

JAYPEE BROTHERS MEDICAL PUBLISHERS
The Health Sciences Publisher
New Delhi | London

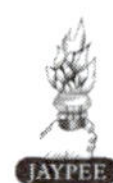

Jaypee Brothers Medical Publishers (P) Ltd

Headquarters
EMCA House
23/23-B, Ansari Road, Daryaganj
New Delhi 110 002, India
Landline: +91-11-23272143, +91-11-23272703
+91-11-23282021, +91-11-23245672
E-mail: jaypee@jaypeebrothers.com

Corporate Office
Jaypee Brothers Medical Publishers (P) Ltd.
4838/24, Ansari Road, Daryaganj
New Delhi 110 002, India
Phone: +91-11-43574357
Fax: +91-11-43574314
E-mail: jaypee@jaypeebrothers.com

Overseas Office
JP Medical Ltd.
83, Victoria Street, London
SW1H 0HW (UK)
Phone: +44-20 3170 8910
E-mail: info@jpmedpub.com

EU GPSR Authorised Representative
Logos Europe, 9 rue Nicolas Poussin
17000, La Rochelle, France
Phone: +33 (0) 6 67 93 73 78
E-mail: Contact@logoseurope.eu

Website: www.jaypeebrothers.com

Website: www.jaypeedigital.com

Inquiries for bulk sales may be solicited at: jaypee@jaypeebrothers.com

Pharmacological Classification of Drugs with Doses and Preparations

First Edition: 1986, Second Edition: 1990, Third Edition: 2006, Fourth Edition: 2010, Fifth Edition: 2014, Sixth Edition: 2019, *Seventh Edition:* **2025**

Reprint: **2026**

ISBN 978-93-6616-559-2

Printed in India by K.K. Printers, Kundli, Haryana-131 028.

Preface

A systematized listing of drugs according to their primary actions, mechanisms, chemical nature, clinical uses and/or other relevant criteria is the first step to learn about them. The mental exercise to prescribe a drug for a patient starts with identifying the class of drugs to be prescribed and then selecting the specific member most appropriate for that patient according to its subclass/group/individual characteristic. For example, the first thing one decides is whether an analgesic or an antihypertensive or an antibiotic is to be prescribed; then proceeds to consider which type of analgesic (opioid/nonopioid), or antihypertensive (calcium channel blocker/angiotensin receptor blocker, etc.), or antibiotic (β-lactam/fluoroquinolone, etc.) is required and then which specific member is most suitable. On the other hand, every drug is known by the class and subclass, to which it belongs, e.g. furosemide is a high-ceiling diuretic, glibenclamide is a sulfonylurea antidiabetic. As such, drug classifications are pivotal to pharmacology students and greatly helpful to prescribing doctors. The phenomenal increase in the number of drugs in recent years has further underscored the need for their logical grouping.

Drug classifications have been criticised for being imprecise and arbitrary because of nonuniform criteria that have often to be adopted and frequent lack of watertight distinctions among drug groups/subgroups. Nevertheless, basing on pharmacological differences and applying appropriate criteria, meaningful drug classifications can be devised. Though, any drug has multiple actions/properties, it can be designated by the most outstanding one. For example, labelling atenolol as a cardioselective β blocker summarises its actions, uses, etc. This booklet has adopted such a pragmatic approach and presented drug classifications that have practical utility. The drug classifications are presented in the form of charts with groups and subgroups of drugs arranged hierarchically. These charts create pictorial images and help memorizing. In this edition all classifications have been updated, expanded and modified where necessary. New drugs, particularly those marketed recently, have been included.

To be useful to medical/pharmacy students as well as to practitioners, the doses (including pediatric doses wherever relevant), frequency and route(s) of administration along with leading brand names of drugs and different types of dosage forms (oral, parenteral, topical, etc.) are listed distinctively after each class of drugs. Thus, essential prescribing information is incorporated for drugs that are available. Single drug formulations are mainly mentioned. Combined drug formulations find a place wherever important or relevant. The listing of brand names is restricted to only 1–4 per drug, and is not exhaustive. Synonyms and alternative names of drugs and classes of drugs are also mentioned. Two separate indices, one of nonproprietary (generic) names and the other of proprietary (brand) names of drugs is provided for instantaneous location of the drug or the product one is looking for.

The present user-friendly format of the booklet is intended to make it a better aid for remembering drug names, identifying the class and subclass to which they belong, and provide easy access to core prescribing information. The credit for meticulous production of this booklet goes to the staff of M/s Jaypee Brothers.

KD Tripathi

Explanatory Notes

1. The information on dosage form(s) is printed in blue colour, and the proprietary (brand) names of drugs/products appear in capital letters.
2. The doses and regimens are given in smaller type, while nonproprietary (generic) drug names appear in bigger type and different font.
3. If no brand name of a drug is listed, it is not currently marketed in India, or is marketed only in combinations. This can be found out from the composition of the combined formulations given.
4. If the route of administration is not specified, the drug is administered orally, and the dose mentioned is the oral dose.
5. Drug doses mentioned without specifying frequency of administration indicate the quantity for a single dose.

Abbreviations

amp	Ampoule
AP	Action potential
BD	Twice daily
BHP	Benign hypertrophy of prostate
BSA	Body surface area
cap	Capsule
CBS	Colloidal bismuth subcitrate
Ch	Child dose
cm	Centimeter
CR	Continuous release
Distab	Dispersible tablet
DS	Double strength
e.c.	Enteric coated
ER	Extended release
ERP	Effective refractory period
ext	Extract
g	Gram
GITS	Gastrointestinal therapeutic system
hr	hour
i.d.	Intradermal
i.m.	Intramuscular
inj	Injection
IU	International unit
i.v.	intravenous
kg	Kilogram
L	Litre
LES	Lower esophageal sphincter
liq	Liquid
m	Meter
max	Maximum
mEq	Milliequivalent
mg	Milligram
min	Minute
ml	Millilitre
MR	Modified release
MU	Mega (million) unit
MW	Molecular weight
μg	Microgram
OD	Once daily
oint	Ointment

Pot.	Potassium
QID	Four times a day
rDNA	Recombinant deoxyribonucleic acid
s.c.	Subcutaneous
s.l.	Sublingual
Sod	Sodium
SR	Sustained release
susp	Suspension
syr	Syrup
tab	Tablet
$TCID_{50}$	Tissue culture infective dose 50%
TDS	Three times a day
THFA	Tetrahydrofolic acid
TTS	Transdermal therapeutic system
U	Unit
UV	Ultra violet
yr	Year (age)
ZE	Zollinger-Ellison

Contents

Drugs Acting on Autonomic Nervous System

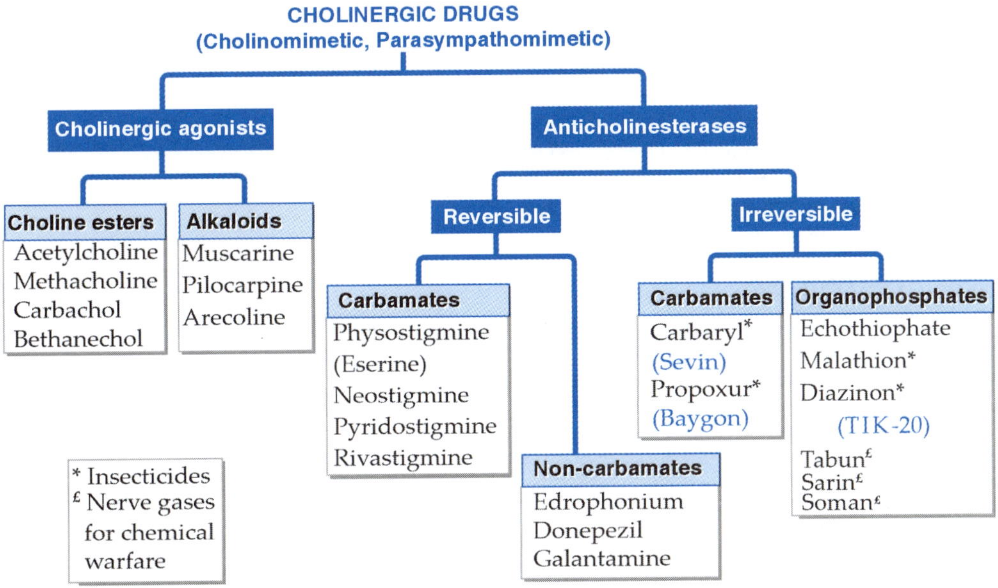

CHOLINERGIC DRUGS
(Cholinomimetic, Parasympathomimetic)

- **Cholinergic agonists**
  - **Choline esters**
    - Acetylcholine
    - Methacholine
    - Carbachol
    - Bethanechol
  - **Alkaloids**
    - Muscarine
    - Pilocarpine
    - Arecoline
- **Anticholinesterases**
  - **Reversible**
    - **Carbamates**
      - Physostigmine (Eserine)
      - Neostigmine
      - Pyridostigmine
      - Rivastigmine
    - **Non-carbamates**
      - Edrophonium
      - Donepezil
      - Galantamine
  - **Irreversible**
    - **Carbamates**
      - Carbaryl* (Sevin)
      - Propoxur* (Baygon)
    - **Organophosphates**
      - Echothiophate
      - Malathion*
      - Diazinon* (TIK-20)
      - Tabun£
      - Sarin£
      - Soman£

* Insecticides
£ Nerve gases for chemical warfare

Preparations

1. **Bethanechol:** 25 mg oral, 2.5–5 mg s.c.
   UROTONE, BETHACOL 25 mg tab.
2. **Pilocarpine:** 0.5–4% topically in eye.
   PILOCAR 1%, 2%, 4% eye drops; CARPINE 0.5% eye drops; PILODROPS 2% eye drops.
3. **Physostigmine:** 0.5–1.0 mg oral/i.m., 0.25–0.5% topically in eye.
   BI-MIOTIC physostigmine 0.25% + pilocarpine nitrate 2% eye drops.
4. **Neostigmine:** 15–30 mg oral, 0.5–2.5 mg s.c./i.m.
   PROSTIGMIN, MYOSTIGMIN, TILSTIGMIN 15 mg tab, 0.5 mg/ml in 1 ml and 5 ml inj.
5. **Pyridostigmine:** 60–120 mg oral 2–3 times a day.
   DISTINON, MYESTIN 60 mg tab.
6. **Edrophonium:** 2–10 mg i.v. or i.m.
   EDROPHONIUM CHLORIDE 10 mg in 1 ml inj.
7. **Rivastigmine:** Initially 1.5 mg BD, increase every 2 weeks by 1.5 mg/day upto 6 mg BD.
   EXELON, RIVAMER 1.5, 3, 4.5, 6.0 mg caps.
8. **Donepezil:** 5 mg at bed time once daily (max 10 mg/day).
   DONECEPT, DOPEZIL, DORENT 5, 10 mg tabs.
9. **Galantamine:** 4 mg BD (max 12 mg BD).
   GALAMER 4, 8, 12 mg tabs.

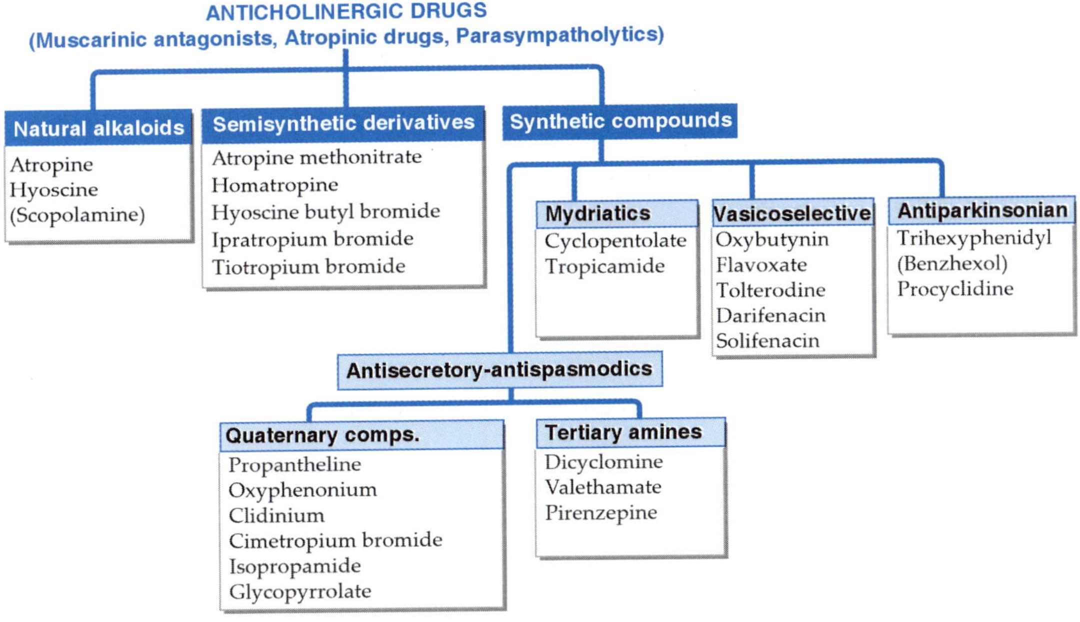
ANTICHOLINERGIC DRUGS
(Muscarinic antagonists, Atropinic drugs, Parasympatholytics)
Natural alkaloids
Atropine
Hyoscine
(Scopolamine)
Semisynthetic derivatives
Atropine methonitrate
Homatropine
Hyoscine butyl bromide
Ipratropium bromide
Tiotropium bromide
Synthetic compounds
Mydriatics
Cyclopentolate
Tropicamide
Vasicoselective
Oxybutynin
Flavoxate
Tolterodine
Darifenacin
Solifenacin
Antiparkinsonian
Trihexyphenidyl
(Benzhexol)
Procyclidine
Antisecretory-antispasmodics
Quaternary comps.
Propantheline
Oxyphenonium
Clidinium
Cimetropium bromide
Isopropamide
Glycopyrrolate
Tertiary amines
Dicyclomine
Valethamate
Pirenzepine

Preparations

1. **Atropine:** 0.6–2.0 mg i.m./i.v. (Child 10 μg/kg), 1–2% topically in eye.
   ATROPINE SULPHATE 0.6 mg/ml inj, ATRO 1% eye drop/oint, ATROSULPH 1% eye drop, 5% eye oint.
2. **Hyoscine hydrobromide:** 0.3–0.5 mg oral/i.m. (Child 10 μg/kg).
3. **Hyoscine butyl bromide:** 20–40 mg oral/i.m./s.c./i.v.
   BUSCOPAN 10 mg tab, 20 mg/ml amp.
4. **Atropine methonitrate:** 2.5–10 mg oral/i.m.
5. **Propantheline:** 15–30 mg oral.
6. **Oxyphenonium:** 5–10 mg (Child 3–5 mg) oral. ANTRENYL 5, 10 mg tab.
7. **Clidinium:** 2.5–5 mg oral.
   In SPASRIL, ARWIN 2.5 mg tab with chlordiazepoxide 5 mg. NORMAXIN, CIBIS 2.5 mg with dicyclomine 10 mg and chlordiazepoxide 5 mg tab.
8. **Cimetropium bromide:** 50 mg 2–3 times a day.
   IBSCIM 50 mg tab.
9. **Isopropamide:** 5 mg oral. In STELABID, GASTABID 5 mg tab. with trifluoperazine 1 mg.
10. **Dicyclomine:** 20 mg oral/i.m.
    CYCLOPAM INJ. 10 mg/ml in 2 ml, 10 ml, 30 ml amp/vial, also 20 mg tab with paracetamol 500 mg; in COLIMEX, 20 mg with paracetamol 500 mg tab.
11. **Valethamate:** 8 mg i.m., 10 mg oral, repeated as required.
    VALAMATE 8 mg in 1 ml inj, EPIDOSIN 10 mg tab, 8 mg inj.
12. **Glycopyrrolate:** 0.2–0.4 mg i.m./i.v., 1–2 mg oral, 25–50 μg by inhalation once daily.
    GLYCO-P 0.2 mg/ml amp., 1 mg in 5 ml vial, PYROLATE 0.2 mg/ml, 1 ml amp, 10 ml vial.
    GLYCOHALE: inhalation solution as 25 μg respules.

13. **Ipratropium bromide:** 40–80 μg by inhalation/nasal spray.
IPRAVENT 20 μg/puff metered dose inhaler, 2 puffs 3–4 times daily; 250 μg/ml respirator soln., 0.4–2 ml nebulized in conjunction with a β_2 agonist 2–4 times daily.
Also used to control rhinorrhoea in perennial rhinitis and common cold; IPRANASE–AQ 0.084% nasal spray (42 μg per actuation), 1–2 sprays in each nostril 3–4 times a day.
14. **Tiotropium bromide:** 18 μg by inhalation. TIOVA 18 μg rotacaps, 1 rotacap by inhalation OD.
15. **Oxybutynin:** 5 mg BD/TDS oral; children above 5 yr 2.5 mg BD.
OXYBUTIN, CYSTRAN, OXYSPAS 2.5 mg and 5 mg tabs.
16. **Flavoxate:** 200 mg TDS. URISPAS, FLAVATE, FLAVOSPAS 200 mg tab.
17. **Tolterodine:** 1–2 mg BD or 2–4 mg OD of sustained release tab. oral; ROLITEN, TOLTER 1, 2 mg tabs, TORQ 2, 4 mg SR tab.
18. **Darifenacin:** 7.5–15 mg once daily; DARILONG, VESIGARD 7.5 mg, 15 mg ER tab.
19. **Solifenacin:** 5–10 mg once daily; SOLICEPT, BISPEC 5, 10 mg tabs.
20. **Homatropine:** 1–2% topically in eye. HOMATROPINE EYE, HOMIDE 1%, 2% eye drops.
21. **Cyclopentolate:** 0.5–1.0% topically in eye.
CYCLOMID EYE, CYCLOGYL, CYCLOPENT 1% eye drops.
22. **Tropicamide:** 0.5–1.0% topically in eye. OPTIMIDE, TROPICAMET, TROMIDE 0.5%, 1% eye drops; TROPAC-P, TROPICAMET PLUS 0.8% + phenylephrine 5% eye drops.
23. **Trihexyphenidyl (benzhexol):** 2–10 mg/day; PACITANE, PARKIN 2 mg tab.
24. **Procyclidine:** 5–20 mg/day; MODIN 2.5, 5 mg tab.

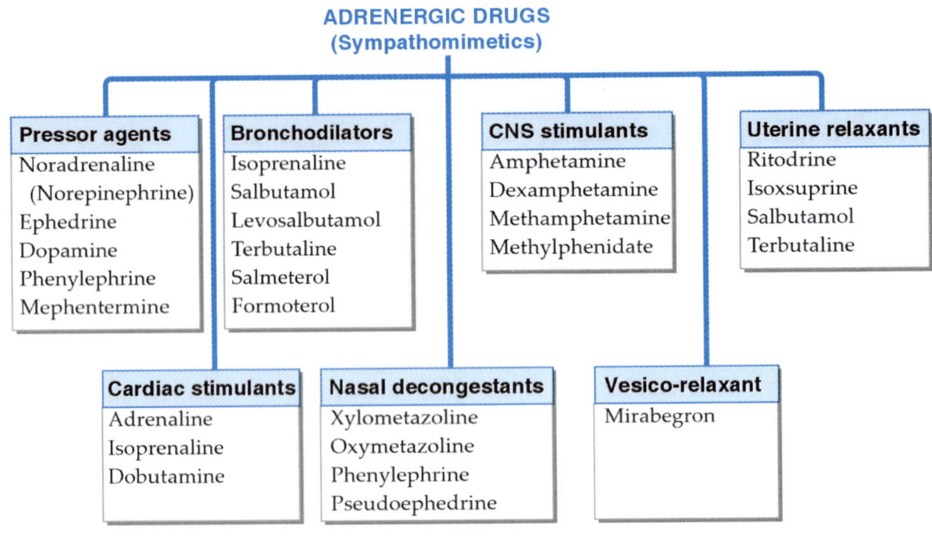
ADRENERGIC DRUGS
(Sympathomimetics)
Pressor agents
Noradrenaline
(Norepinephrine)
Ephedrine
Dopamine
Phenylephrine
Mephentermine
Bronchodilators
Isoprenaline
Salbutamol
Levosalbutamol
Terbutaline
Salmeterol
Formoterol
CNS stimulants
Amphetamine
Dexamphetamine
Methamphetamine
Methylphenidate
Uterine relaxants
Ritodrine
Isoxsuprine
Salbutamol
Terbutaline
Cardiac stimulants
Adrenaline
Isoprenaline
Dobutamine
Nasal decongestants
Xylometazoline
Oxymetazoline
Phenylephrine
Pseudoephedrine
Vesico-relaxant
Mirabegron

Preparations

1. **Adrenaline (Epinephrine):** 0.2–0.5 mg s.c./i.m.;
   ADRENALINE 1 mg/ml inj; ADRENA 4 mg (of adrenaline bitartrate=2 mg adrenaline base) per 2 ml inj.
2. **Noradrenaline (Norepinephrine, Levarterenol):** 2–4 μg/min i.v. infusion;
   ADRENOR, NORAD 2 mg (base)/2 ml amp.
3. **Isoprenaline (Isoproterenol):** 20 mg s.l., 1–2 mg i.m., 5–10 μg/min i.v. infusion;
   NEOEPININE 20 mg sublingual tab, ISOPRIN, ISOSOL 4 mg/2 ml inj.
4. **Dopamine:** 0.2–1.0 mg/min i.v. infusion; DOPAMINE, DOPACARD 200 mg/5 ml amp, to be diluted in saline and infused i.v.
5. **Dobutamine:** 2–8 μg/kg/min i.v. infusion;
   CARDIJECT 50 mg/4 ml and 250 mg/20 ml inj, DOBUTREX, DOBUSTAT 250 mg vial.
6. **Ephedrine:** 15–60 mg oral, 15–30 mg i.m./i.v.;
   SULFIDRIN 50 mg in 1 ml inj.
7. **Phenylephrine:** 5–10 mg oral, 2–5 mg i.m., 0.1–0.5 mg slow i.v. inj, 30–60 μg/min i.v. infusion, 5–10% topically in eye; in DECOLD PLUS 5 mg with paracetamol 400 mg + chlorpheniramine 2 mg + caffeine 15 mg tab; SOLVIN COLD. 10 mg with chlorpheniramine 2 mg, paracetamol 500 mg tab; FRENIN 10 mg in 1 ml inj, DROSYN 10% eye drops, in DROSYN-T, TROPAC-P 5% with tropicamide 0.8% eye drops.
8. **Mephentermine:** 10–20 mg oral/i.m., also by i.v. infusion.
   MEPHENTINE 10 mg tab, 15 mg in 1 ml amp, 30 mg/ml in 10 ml vial, TERMIN 30 mg/ml in 10 ml vial.
9. **Amphetamine:** 5–15 mg oral.
10. **Dexamphetamine:** 5–10 mg (children 2.5–5 mg) oral.
11. **Methamphetamine:** 5–10 mg oral.

12. **Methylphenidate:** 5–10 mg BD for adults; children 0.25 mg/kg/day.
RETALIN 5, 10, 20 mg tab. (availability restricted).
13. **Xylometazoline:** 0.05%–0.1% topically in nose;
OTRIVIN 0.05% (pediatric), 0.1% (adult) nasal drops and nasal spray, OTRINOZ 0.025%, 0.05%, 0.1% nasal drops.
14. **Oxymetazoline:** 0.025–0.05% topically in nose;
NASIVION, OTRIVIN OXY, SINAREST 0.025% (pediatric), 0.05% (adult) nasal drops, RHINOJET 0.05% nasal spray.
15. **Pseudoephedrine:** 30–60 mg oral TDS.
SOLVIN OD: pseudoephedrine 120 mg + levocetirizine 5 mg SR tab.
16. **Ritodrine:** 50–200 μg/min i.v. infusion, 10 mg i.m./oral 4–6 hourly; YUTOPAR, RITROD 10 mg/ml inj (5 ml amp), 10 mg tab. RITODINE 10 mg tab, 10 mg in 1 ml inj.
17. **Isoxsuprine:** 5–10 mg oral, i.m. 4–6 hourly, DUVADILAN 10 mg tab, 40 mg SR cap, 10 mg/2 ml inj.
18. **Mirabegron:** 25–50 mg once daily as extended release tab.
MIRAGO 25, 50 mg SR tab; MIRBEG, EXENA 25 mg ER tab.

Note: For doses and preparations of β_2 agonist bronchodilators (salbutamol, etc.) *See* p. 33.

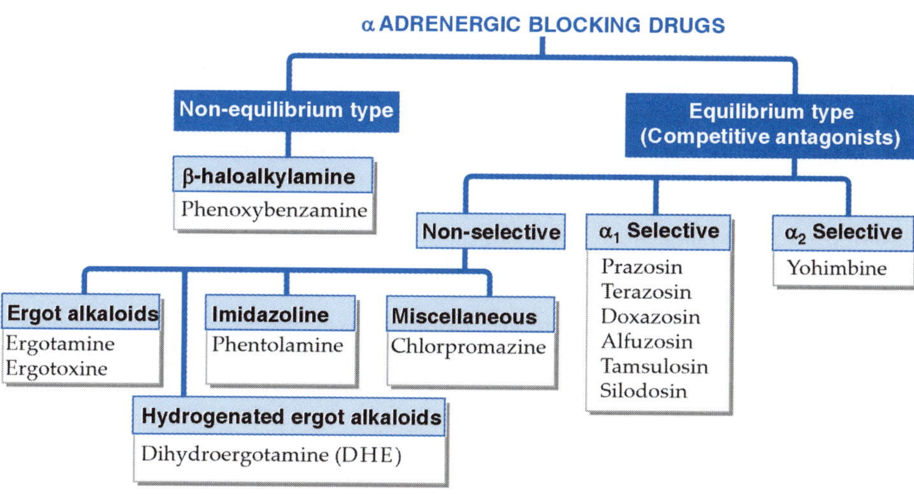
α ADRENERGIC BLOCKING DRUGS
Non-equilibrium type
β-haloalkylamine
Phenoxybenzamine
Equilibrium type (Competitive antagonists)
Non-selective
α1 Selective
Prazosin
Terazosin
Doxazosin
Alfuzosin
Tamsulosin
Silodosin
α2 Selective
Yohimbine
Ergot alkaloids
Ergotamine
Ergotoxine
Imidazoline
Phentolamine
Miscellaneous
Chlorpromazine
Hydrogenated ergot alkaloids
Dihydroergotamine (DHE)

Preparations

1. **Phenoxybenzamine:** 20–60 mg/day oral, 1 mg/kg slow i.v. infusion over 1 hour; FENOXENE 10 mg cap, 50 mg/ml inj, BIOPHENOX 50 mg/ml inj.
2. **Ergotamine:** For migraine 1–3 mg oral/sublingual, repeat as required (max 6 mg in a day); rarely 0.25–0.5 mg i.m. or s.c.; MIGRIL: Ergotamine 2 mg, caffeine 100 mg, cyclizine 50 mg tab. VASOGRAIN: Ergotamine 1 mg, caffeine 100 mg, paracetamol 250 mg, prochlorperazine 2.5 mg tab.
3. **Dihydroergotamine:** For migraine 2–6 mg oral, 0.5–1 mg i.m., s.c. repeat hourly (max 3 mg).
4. **Phentolamine:** 5 mg i.v. repeated as required; FENTANOR 10 mg/ml inj.
5. **Prazosin:** Start with 0.5–1 mg at bedtime; usual dose 1–4 mg BD or TDS; PRAZOPRES 1.0 and 2.0 mg tabs. MINIPRESS XL: Prazosin GITS (gastrointestinal therapeutic system) 2.5 mg and 5 mg tablets; 1 tab OD.
6. **Terazosin:** Usual maintenance dose 2–5 mg OD; HYTRIN, TERALFA, OLYSTER 1, 2, 5 mg tab.
7. **Doxazosin:** 1 mg OD initially, increase upto 4 mg BD; DOXACARD, DURACARD, DOXAPRESS 1, 2 mg tabs.
8. **Alfuzosin:** 2.5 BD-QID or 10 mg OD as extended release tab. ALFUSIN, ALFOO 10 mg ER tab.
9. **Tamsulosin:** URIMAX, DYNAPRES 0.2, 0.4 mg MR cap; CONTIFLO-OD 0.4 mg cap; 1 cap (max 2) in the morning with meals.
10. **Silodosin:** 4–8 mg OD; RAPILIF, SILODAL 4, 8 mg cap.
11. **Yohimbine:** 2 mg oral.

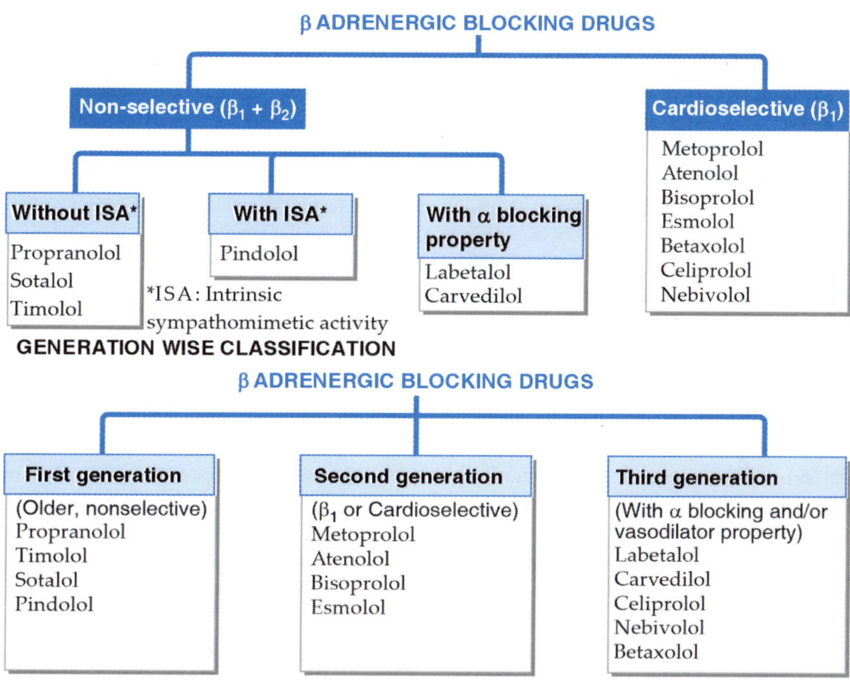
β ADRENERGIC BLOCKING DRUGS
Non-selective (β1 + β2)
Cardioselective (β1)
Metoprolol
Atenolol
Bisoprolol
Esmolol
Betaxolol
Celiprolol
Nebivolol
Without ISA*
Propranolol
Sotalol
Timolol
With ISA*
Pindolol
With α blocking property
Labetalol
Carvedilol
*ISA: Intrinsic sympathomimetic activity
GENERATION WISE CLASSIFICATION
β ADRENERGIC BLOCKING DRUGS
First generation
(Older, nonselective)
Propranolol
Timolol
Sotalol
Pindolol
Second generation
(β1 or Cardioselective)
Metoprolol
Atenolol
Bisoprolol
Esmolol
Third generation
(With α blocking and/or vasodilator property)
Labetalol
Carvedilol
Celiprolol
Nebivolol
Betaxolol

Preparations

1. Propranolol: Oral—10 mg BD to 160 mg QID (average 40–160 mg/day). Start with a low dose and gradually increase according to need; i.v.—2 to 5 mg injected over 10 min with constant monitoring.
   CIPLAR-LA 10 mg, 40 mg long acting tab, INDERAL, CIPLAR, BETABLOC 10, 40 mg tab.
2. Sotalol: 80 mg BD–160 mg TDS oral; SOTAGARD 40, 80 mg tabs.
3. Pindolol: 5–15 mg BD; VISKEN 10, 15 mg tab.
4. Metoprolol: 25 mg BD–100 mg QID oral, 5–15 mg slow i.v. inj;
   BETALOC 25, 50, 100 mg tab, LOPRESOR, METOLAR XR 25, 50, 100 mg tab.
5. S(–) Metoprolol: 12.5–50 mg BD; METPURE–XL 12.5, 25, 50 mg ER tabs.
6. Atenolol: 25 mg OD–50 mg BD; BETACARD, ATEN, TENORMIN 25, 50, 100 mg tabs.
7. S(–) Atenolol: 12.5–50 mg OD; ATPURE 12.5, 25, 50 mg tabs.
8. Bisoprolol: 2.5–10 mg OD; CONCOR, CORBIS 5 mg tab.
9. Esmolol: 0.5 mg/kg i.v. injection followed by 0.05–0.2 mg/kg/min i.v. infusion;
   MINIBLOCK 100 mg/10 ml, 250 mg/10 ml inj.
10. Celiprolol: 100 mg OD–300 mg BD; CELICARD 200 mg tab.
11. Nebivolol: 5 mg OD (start with 2.5 mg OD in elderly); NODON 5 mg tab, NEBICARD 2.5, 5 mg tabs.
12. Labetalol: Start with 50 mg BD, increase to 100–200 mg TDS oral. In hypertensive emergencies 20–40 mg slow i.v. injection every 10 min till desired response is obtained (max. 300 mg).
    NORMADATE 50, 100, 200 mg tab; LABECOR 100 mg tab, LABETA 20 mg/4 ml inj.
13. Carvedilol: *for CHF:* Start with 3.125 mg BD for 2 weeks, if well tolerated, gradually increase to max. of 25 mg BD.
    for hypertension/angina: 6.25 mg BD initially, titrate to max. of 25 mg BD.
    CARVIL, CARLOC, CARVAS 3.125, 6.25, 12.5, 25 mg tabs; ORICAR 12.5, 25 mg tabs.

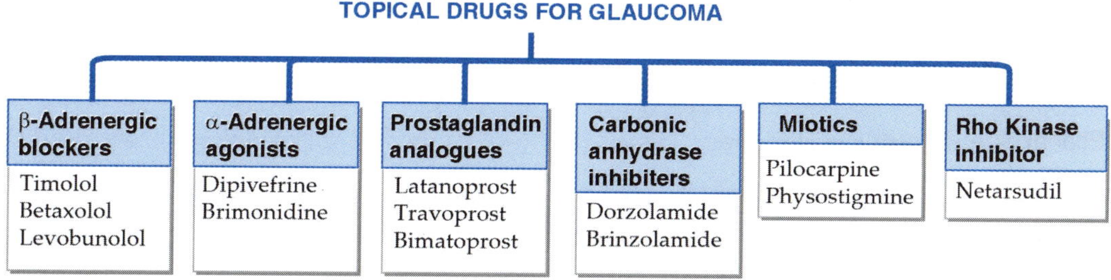

Preparations

1. **Timolol:** Start with 0.25% eye drops BD, change to 0.5% drops in case of inadequate response. 0.5% OD as gel forming solution. GLUCOMOL, OCUPRES, IOTIM, LOPRES 0.25% and 0.5% eye drops, TIMOLAST 0.5% gel forming eye drops (long acting).

   Timolol 0.5% + Latanoprost 0.005%: LAPROST PLUS, LATOCHEK-T eye drops.
2. **Betaxolol:** 0.5% topically in eye BD; IOBET, OCUBETA 0.5% eye drops.
3. **Levobunolol:** 0.5% topically in eye OD; BETAGAN 0.5% ophthalmic solution.
4. **Dipivefrine:** 0.1% topically in eye BD.
5. **Brimonidine:** 0.15%, 0.2% topically in eye TDS;
   ALPHAGAN-P 0.15% eye drops, IOBRIM, BRIMODIN 0.2% eye drops.
6. **Latanoprost:** 0.005% topically in eye OD in evening;
   XALATAN, LATOPROST, 9 PM 50 μg/ml eye drops; LACOMA-T, LAPROST-PLUS, LATOCHEK-T with timolol 0.5% eye drops (store in cold place).

7. **Travoprost:** 0.004% topically in eye OD in evening; TRAVATAN 0.004% eye drops (refrigeration of the eye drops not required); TRAVACOM 0.004% with timolol 0.5% eye drops.
8. **Bimatoprost:** 0.03% as eye drops OD in evening; LUMIGAN, CAREPROST 0.03% eye drops; the eye drop need not be stored in refrigerator; CAREPROST-PLUS, GANFORT with timolol 0.5% eye drop.
9. **Pilocarpine:** 0.5%–4% topically in eye; PILOCAR 1%, 2%, 4% eye drops. CARPINE 0.5% eye drops, PILO DROPS 2% eye drops.
10. **Dorzolamide:** 2% topically in eye BD–TDS; DORTAS, DORZOX 2% eye drops.
11. **Netarsudil:** 0.02% eye drop once daily in evening.
    RHOPRESSA, NETALO 0.02% Ophthalmic solu. (store at 4–8°C).

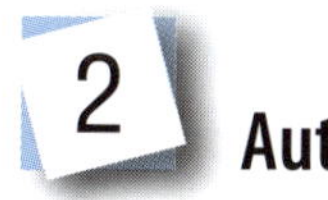

Autacoids and Related Drugs

HISTAMINERGIC AGONISTS

Nonselective agonists ($H_1 + H_2 + H_3$)
- Histamine
- Betahistine

Selective H_1 agonists
- 2-Methyl histamine
- 2-Pyridyl ethylamine
- 2-Thizolyl ethylamine

Selective H_2 agonists
- Dimaprit
- Impromidine

Selective H_3 agonists
- (R) α-Methylhistamine
- Imetit

H_1 ANTAGONISTS (Antihistaminics)

First generation (conventional)

Highly sedative
- Diphenhydramine
- Dimenhydrinate
- Promethazine
- Hydroxyzine

Moderately sedative
- Pheniramine
- Cyproheptadine
- Meclozine
- Cinnarizine

Mildly sedative
- Chlorpheniramine
- Dexchlorpheniramine
- Triprolidine
- Clemastine

Second generation
- Loratadine
- Cetirizine
- Azelastine
- Mizolastine
- Ebastine
- Rupatadine

Third generation
- Fexofenadine
- Desloratadine
- Levocetirizine

Preparations

Betahistine (Histaminergic agonist): 4–8 mg 6–8 hourly; VERTIN 8 mg tab.

1. Diphenhydramine: 25–50 mg oral; BENADRYL 25 mg cap, 12.5 mg/5 ml syr.
2. Dimenhydrinate: 25–50 mg oral; DRAMAMINE 16 mg/5 ml syr, 50 mg tab, GRAVOL 50 mg tab.
3. Promethazine: 25–50 mg oral, i.m. (1 mg/kg); PHENERGAN 10, 25 mg tab, 5 mg/ml elixir, 25 mg/ml inj.
4. Hydroxyzine: 25–50 mg oral, i.m.; ATARAX 10, 25 mg tab, 10 mg/5 ml syr, 6 mg/ml drops, 25 mg/ml inj.
5. Pheniramine: 25–50 mg oral, i.m.; AVIL 25 mg, 50 mg tab, 15 mg/5 ml syr, 22.5 mg/ml inj.
6. Cyproheptadine: 4 mg oral; PRACTIN, CIPLACTIN 4 mg tab., 2 mg/5 ml syrup.
7. Meclozine (Meclizine): 25–50 mg oral;
   In DILIGAN 12.5 mg + niacin 50 mg tab., In PREGNIDOXIN 25 mg + Caffeine 20 mg tab.
8. Cinnarizine: 25–50 mg oral; STUGERON, VERTIGON 25 mg and 75 mg tab.
9. Chlorpheniramine: 2–4 mg (0.1 mg/kg) oral, i.m.; PIRITON, CADISTIN 4 mg tab.
10. Dexchlorpheniramine: 2 mg oral; POLARAMINE 2 mg tab., 0.5 mg/5 ml syrup.
11. Triprolidine: 2.5–5 mg oral; ACTIDIL 2.5 mg tab.
12. Clemastine: 1–2 mg oral; TAVEGYL 1 mg tab., 0.5 mg/5 ml syr.
13. Fexofenadine: 120–180 mg oral; ALLEGRA, ALTIVA, FEXO 120 mg, 180 mg tab.
14. Loratadine: 10 mg oral; LORFAST, LORIDIN, LORMEG, 10 mg tab, 1 mg/ml susp.
15. Desloratadine: 5–10 mg oral; DESLOR, LORDAY, NEOLORIDIN 5 mg tab, DAZIT 10 mg tab.
16. Cetirizine: 10 mg oral; ALERID, CETZINE, ZIRTIN, SIZON 10 mg tab, 5 mg/5 ml syr.
17. Levocetirizine: 5–10 mg oral; LEVORID, LEVOSIZ 5 mg, 10 mg tab, TECZINE 5, 10 mg tab, LEVOCET 5 mg tab, 2.5 mg/5 ml syr. RHINOSOLVIN: Levocetirizine 5 mg + montelukast 10 mg tab.

18. **Azelastine:** 4 mg oral, 0.28 mg intranasal; AZEP NASAL SPRAY 0.14 mg per puff nasal spray.
19. **Mizolastine:** 10 mg oral; ELINA 10 mg tab.
20. **Ebastine:** 10 mg oral; EBAST 10 mg tab.
21. **Rupatadine:** 10 mg oral; RUPAHIST 10 mg tab.

Note: For H_2-Antagonists (H_2-Antihistaminics) *See* p. 129, 130.

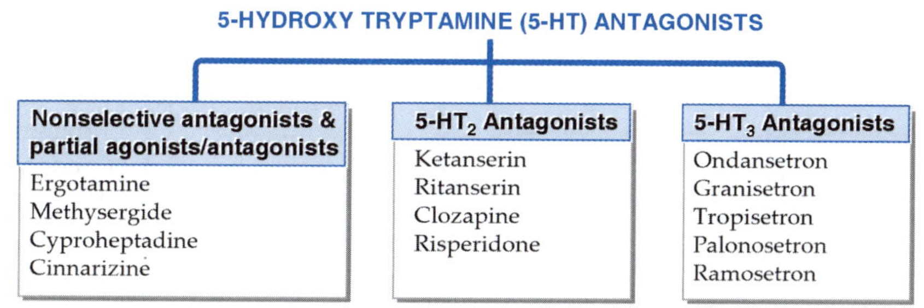

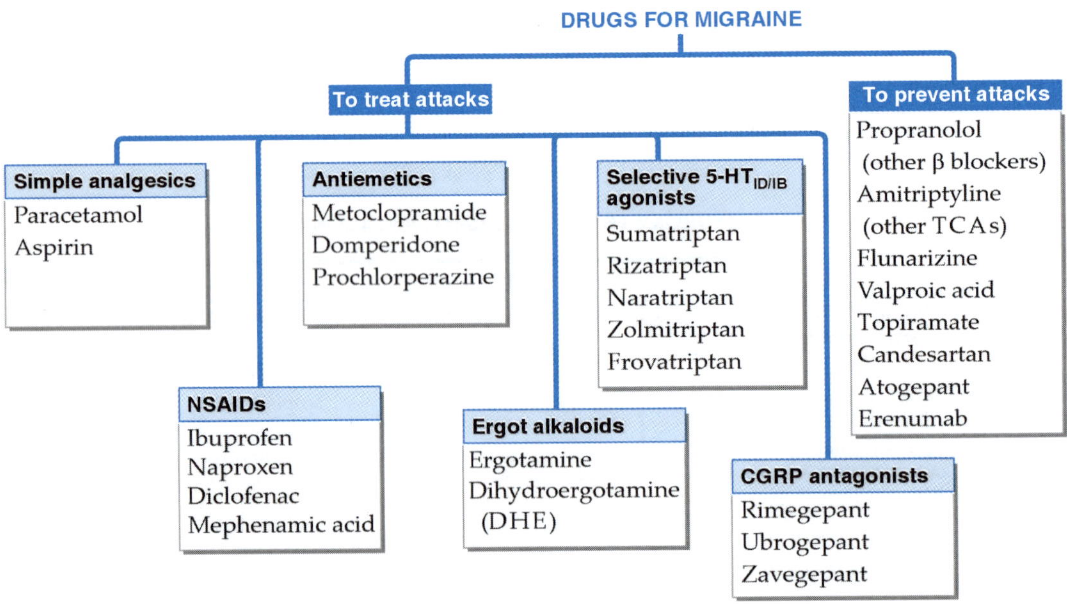
DRUGS FOR MIGRAINE
To treat attacks
To prevent attacks
Propranolol
(other β blockers)
Amitriptyline
(other TCAs)
Flunarizine
Valproic acid
Topiramate
Candesartan
Atogepant
Erenumab
Simple analgesics
Paracetamol
Aspirin
Antiemetics
Metoclopramide
Domperidone
Prochlorperazine
Selective 5-HT$_{ID/IB}$ agonists
Sumatriptan
Rizatriptan
Naratriptan
Zolmitriptan
Frovatriptan
NSAIDs
Ibuprofen
Naproxen
Diclofenac
Mephenamic acid
Ergot alkaloids
Ergotamine
Dihydroergotamine
(DHE)
CGRP antagonists
Rimegepant
Ubrogepant
Zavegepant

Preparations

1. **Ergotamine:** 1 mg oral/sublingual, repeat as required (max. 6 mg), 0.25–0.5 mg s.c./i.m.;
   ERGOTAMINE 1 mg tab.
   MIGRIL: Ergotamine 2 mg, caffeine 100 mg, cyclizine 50 mg tab.
   VASOGRAIN: Ergotamine 1 mg, caffeine 100 mg, paracetamol 250 mg, prochlorperazine 2.5 mg tab.
2. **Dihydroergotamine (DHE):** 2–6 mg oral (max. 10 mg/day), 0.5–1.0 mg i.m., s.c.
3. **Sumatriptan:** 6 mg s.c., 50–100 mg oral at the onset of migraine attack, may be repeated once within 24 hours if required. Those not responding to the first dose should not be given the second dose; 25 mg nasal spray, may be repeated once after 2 hours;
   SUMINAT, SUMITREX 25, 50, 100 mg tabs, 25 mg nasal spray, 6 mg/0.5 ml inj. MIGRATAN 50, 100 mg tabs.
4. **Rizatriptan:** 5-10 mg at the onset of migraine attack, may be repeated after 2 hours if required.Those not responding to the first dose should not be given the second dose; RIZACT, RIZATAN 5 mg, 10 mg tabs.
5. **Naratriptan:** 2.5 mg oral; NARATREX 2.5 mg tab.
6. **Frovatriptan:** 2.5 mg oral; FROVA 2.5 mg tab.
7. **Zolmitriptan:** 2.5-5 mg oral; 5 mg by nasal spray; ZOMING 2.5 mg, 5 mg tabs, ZOLMIST 5 mg nasal spray.
8. **Rimegepant:** 75 mg oral; NURTEC 75 mg oral dissolving tab., only 1 tab to be taken in 24 hr.
9. **Atogepant:** 30–60 mg OD; QULIPTA 10, 30, 60 mg tab.
10. **Flunarizine:** 10–20 mg OD, children 5 mg OD; NOMIGRAIN, FLUNARIN 5 mg, 10 mg caps/tab.

Note: For preparations of other drugs, *see* Index.

PROSTAGLANDINS (PGs)

Natural prostaglandins

- Dinoprostone (PGE_2)
- Gemeprost
- Dinoprost ($PGF_{2\alpha}$)
- Alprostadil (PGE_1)
- Prostacyclin (PGI_2) (Epoprostenol)

Prostaglandin analogues

- Carboprost (15-methyl $PGF_{2\alpha}$)
- Misoprostol (methyl PGE_1 ester)
- Latanoprost ($PGF_{2\alpha}$ analogue)
- Travoprost
- Bimatoprost

Preparations

1. **PGE$_2$ (Dinoprostone):** PROSTIN-E$_2$ for induction/augmentation of labour, midterm abortion.
   Vaginal gel (1 mg or 2 mg in 2.5 ml) 1 mg inserted into posterior fornix, followed by 1–2 mg after 6 hour if required.
   Vaginal tab (3 mg) 3 mg inserted into posterior fornix, followed by another 3 mg if labour does not start within 6 hour.
   Extraamniotic solution (10 mg/ml in 0.5 ml amp.) infrequently used.
   Oral tablet PRIMIPROST 0.5 mg tab, one tab. hourly till induction, max 1.5 mg per hr; rarely used.
   Cervical gel CERVIPRIME (0.5 mg in 2.5 ml prefilled syringe) 0.5 mg inserted into cervical canal for preinduction cervical softening and dilatation in patients with poor Bishop's score.
2. **Gemeprost:** CERVAGEM 1 mg vaginal pessary: for softening of cervix in first trimester–1 mg 3 hr before attempting dilatation; for 2nd trimester abortion/molar gestation—1 mg every 3 hours, max. 5 doses.
3. **PGF$_{2\alpha}$ (Dinoprost):** PROSTIN F$_2$ ALPHA intraamniotic injection, 5 mg/ml in 4 ml amp. for midterm abortion/induction of labour (rarely used).
4. **15-methyl PGF$_{2\alpha}$ (Carboprost):** PROSTODIN 0.25 mg in 1 ml amp; 0.25 mg i.m. every 30–120 min for PPH, midterm abortion, missed abortion.
5. **Misoprostol (methyl–PGE$_1$ ester):** MIFEGEST Kit, UNWANTED Kit, MTP Kit: Mifepristone 200 mg (1 tab) + Misoprostol 200 μg (4 tabs); For termination of pregnancy upto 49 days—take mifepristone 1 tab orally, after 24 hours insert misoprostol 4 tabs intravaginally before going to be bed (bleeding starts after 2–6 hours).
6. **PGE$_1$ (Alprostadil):** 0.5 mg by slow i.v. infusion; PROSTIN–VR, BIOGLANDIN 0.5 mg in 1 ml inj.
7. **PGI$_2$ (Prostacyclin, Epoprostenol):** 0.5 mg by i.v. infusion or injection in extracorporeal circulation; FLOLAN 0.5 mg per vial for reconstitution.

Note: For preparations of other analogues, *see* Index.

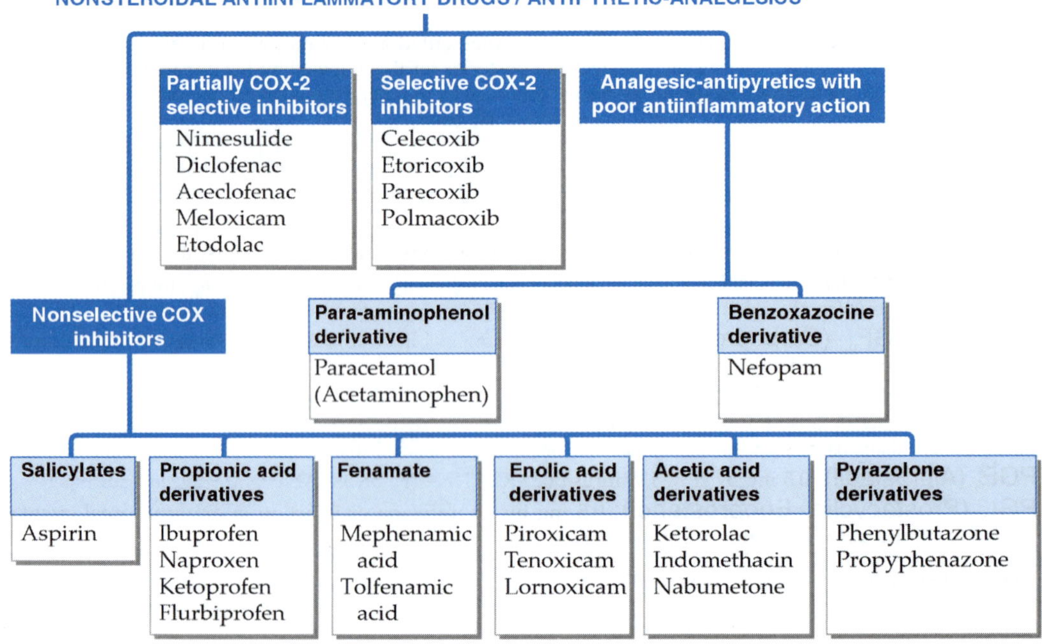
NONSTEROIDAL ANTIINFLAMMATORY DRUGS / ANTIPYRETIC-ANALGESICS
Partially COX-2 selective inhibitors
Nimesulide
Diclofenac
Aceclofenac
Meloxicam
Etodolac
Selective COX-2 inhibitors
Celecoxib
Etoricoxib
Parecoxib
Polmacoxib
Analgesic-antipyretics with poor antiinflammatory action
Nonselective COX inhibitors
Para-aminophenol derivative
Paracetamol (Acetaminophen)
Benzoxazocine derivative
Nefopam
Salicylates
Aspirin
Propionic acid derivatives
Ibuprofen
Naproxen
Ketoprofen
Flurbiprofen
Fenamate
Mephenamic acid
Tolfenamic acid
Enolic acid derivatives
Piroxicam
Tenoxicam
Lornoxicam
Acetic acid derivatives
Ketorolac
Indomethacin
Nabumetone
Pyrazolone derivatives
Phenylbutazone
Propyphenazone

Preparations

1. **Aspirin:** Antiinflammatory dose 3–5 g/day (75–100 mg/kg/day); analgesic-antipyretic dose 0.3–0.6 g 6–8 hourly; antiplatelet dose 75–150 mg/day. ASPIRIN 350 mg tab, COLSPRIN 100, 325 mg tabs, ECOSPRIN 75, 150, 325 mg tabs, DISPRIN 325 mg (with calcium carbonate 105 mg + citric acid 35 mg) tab, LOPRIN 75 mg tab.

   BIOSPIRIN: Lysine acetylsalicylate 900 mg + glycine 100 mg/vial for dissolving in 5 ml water and i.v. injection.
2. **Ibuprofen:** 400–600 mg (5–10 mg/kg) TDS;
   BRUFEN, IBUSYNTH 200, 400, 600 mg tab, IBUGESIC also 100 mg/5 ml susp.
3. **Naproxen:** 250–500 mg BD
   NAPROSYN 250 mg, 500 mg tabs, ARTAGEN, XENOBID 250 mg tab.
4. **Ketoprofen:** 50–100 mg BD–TDS;
   KETOFEN 50, 100 mg tab; OSTOFEN 50 mg cap. RHOFENID 100 mg tab, 200 mg SR tab; 100 mg/2 ml amp.
5. **Flurbiprofen:** 50 mg BD–TDS;
   FLUROFEN 100 mg tab, OCUFLUR 0.03% eye drops.
6. **Mephenamic acid:** 250–500 mg TDS; MEFTAL 250, 500 mg tab, 100 mg/5 ml susp. PONSTAN 125, 250, 500 mg tab, 50 mg/ml syrup.
7. **Tolfenamic acid:** 200 mg BD-TDS; CLOTAN, TOLFEGRAN 200 mg tab.
8. **Diclofenac:** 50–75 mg TDS, oral 75 mg deep i.m.; VOVERAN, DICLONAC, MOVONAC 50 mg enteric coated tab, 100 mg S.R. tab, 25 mg/ml in 3 ml amp. for i.m. inj. DICLOMAX 25, 50 mg tab, 75 mg/3 ml inj, DYNAPAR-AQ, JUSTIN-AQ: Diclofenac sod. 75 mg in 1 ml for i.v. or i.m. inj.

   Diclofenac potassium: VOLTAFLAM 25, 50 mg tab, ULTRA-K 50 mg tab; VOVERAN 1% topical gel, VOVERAN OPHTHA 0.1% eye drops.
9. **Aceclofenac:** 100 mg BD; ACECLO, DOLOKIND, ZERODOL 100 mg tab, 200 mg SR tab.

10. **Piroxicam:** 20 mg BD for two days followed by 20 mg OD; DOLONEX, PIROX 20 mg cap, 20 mg dispersible tab, 20 mg/ml inj in 1 and 2 ml amps; PIRICAM 10, 20 mg caps.
11. **Tenoxicam:** 20 mg OD; TOBITIL 20 mg tab.
12. **Lornoxicam:** 8–16 mg/day in 2–3 divided doses.
    FLEXILOR, XOFEN, LOFECAM, LORSAID 4, 8 mg tabs.
13. **Ketorolac:** 10–20 mg oral 6 hourly, 15–30 mg i.m./i.v. 6 hourly (max 90 mg/day); KETOROL, ZOROVON, KETANOV, TOROLAC 10 mg tab, 30 mg in 1 ml amp., KETLUR, ACULAR 0.5% eye drops.
14. **Indomethacin:** 25–50 mg BD–QID. Those not tolerating the drug orally may be given nightly suppository. IDICIN, INDOCAP 25 mg cap, 75 mg SR cap, ARTICID 25, 50 mg cap, INDOFLAM 25, 75 mg caps, 1% eye drop. RECTICIN 50 mg suppository.
15. **Nimesulide:** 100 mg BD; NIMULID, NIMEGESIC, NIMODOL 100 mg tab.
16. **Meloxicam:** 7.5–15 mg OD; MELFLAM, MEL–OD, MUVIK, M–CAM 7.5 mg, 15 mg tabs.
17. **Nabumetone:** 500 mg OD (max 500 mg BD); NABUFLAM 500 mg tab.
18. **Etodolac:** 200-400 mg BD-TDS; ETOVA 200, 300, 400 mg tabs, ETOGESIC 400 mg tab.
19. **Celecoxib:** 100–200 mg BD; CELACT, COLCIBRA, REVIBRA 100, 200 mg caps.
20. **Etoricoxib:** 60–120 mg OD; TOROCOXIA, ETOXIB, ETOSHINE, NUCOXIA 60, 90, 120 mg tabs.
21. **Polmacoxib:** 2 mg once daily; POLVOLT, POLIEXAR 2 mg cap.
22. **Parecoxib:** 40 mg oral/i.m./i.v. repeated after 6–12 hours (max. 80 mg/day); PAROXIB, REVALDO, VALTO-P 40 mg/vial inj.
23. **Paracetamol:** 325–650 mg (children 10–15 mg/kg) 3-5 times a day (max. 2600 mg/day); also 80–250 mg as suppository in infants and children; CROCIN 0.5 g tab, 125 mg/5 ml and 250 mg/5 ml syr, 100 mg/ml pediatric drops, CROCIN PAIN RELIEF 650 mg with caffeine 50 mg tab; METACIN, PARACIN 500 mg tab, 125 mg/5 ml

syrup, 150 mg/ml ped. drops, ULTRAGIN, PYRIGESIC, CALPOL 500 mg tab, 125 mg/5 ml syrup, NEOMOL, FEVASTIN, FEBRINIL 300 mg/2 ml inj. JUNIMOL-RDS 80, 170, 250 mg suppository, PARACETAMOL RECTAL SUPPOSITORY 80, 170 mg; KABIPARA: Paracetamol 1 g/100 ml for slow i.v. injection, AEKNIL 150 mg/ml inj in 2 ml, 3 ml, 15 ml amps for slow i.v. inj.

24. Nefopam: 30–60 mg TDS oral, 20 mg i.m. 6 hourly; NEFOMAX 30 mg tab, 20 mg in 1 ml amp.

Topical NSAIDs

1. Diclofenac 1% gel: VOLINI GEL, RELAXYL GEL, DICLONAC GEL
2. Ibuprofen 10% gel: RIBUFEN GEL
3. Naproxen 10% gel: NAPROSYN GEL
4. Ketoprofen 2.5% gel: RHOFENID GEL
5. Flurbiprofen 5% gel: FROBEN GEL
6. Nimesulide 1% gel: NIMULID TRANS GEL, NIMEGESIC-T-GEL
7. Piroxicam 0.5% gel: DOLONEX GEL, MOVON GEL, PIROX GEL, MINICAM GEL
8. Aceclofenac 1.5% gel: ZERODOL GEL

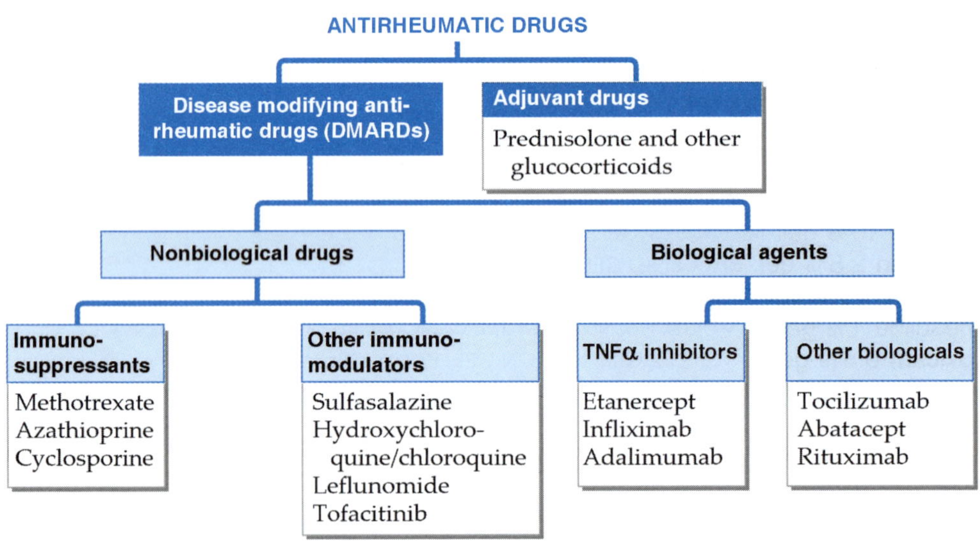
ANTIRHEUMATIC DRUGS
Disease modifying anti-rheumatic drugs (DMARDs)
Adjuvant drugs
Prednisolone and other glucocorticoids
Nonbiological drugs
Biological agents
Immuno-suppressants
Methotrexate
Azathioprine
Cyclosporine
Other immuno-modulators
Sulfasalazine
Hydroxychloro-quine/chloroquine
Leflunomide
Tofacitinib
TNFα inhibitors
Etanercept
Infliximab
Adalimumab
Other biologicals
Tocilizumab
Abatacept
Rituximab

Preparations

1. **Methotrexate:** 7.5–15 mg weekly oral; NEOTREXATE, BIOTREXATE 2.5 mg tab, FOLITREX 2.5 mg, 5 mg, 7.5 mg, 10 mg, 15 mg tabs.
2. **Azathioprine:** 50–150 mg/day; IMURAN, AZORAN, AZOPRINE 50 mg tab.
3. **Sulfasalazine:** 1–3 g/day in 2–3 divided doses; SALAZOPYRIN, SAZO-EN 0.5 g tab.
4. **Chloroquine:** 150 mg (base) per day; LARIAGO, RESOCHIN, NIVAQUIN-P 250 mg as phosphate (150 mg base) tab.
5. **Hydroxychloroquine:** initially 200 mg BD, followed by 200 mg OD for maintenance; ZHQUINE, ZYQ, HCQS 200 mg, 400 mg tabs.
6. **Leflunomide:** 100 mg/day for 3 days loading dose, followed by 20 mg OD; LEFRA 10 mg, 20 mg tabs.
7. **Etanercept:** 25–50 mg s.c. once or twice weekly; ENBREL, ENBROL 25 mg/0.5 ml and 50 mg/1 ml inj.
8. **Tofacitinib:** 5 mg BD; TOFASTAR, TOFZA, TOBRAZA, TFCT-NIB 5 mg tab.
9. **Infliximab:** 3–5 mg/kg infused i.v. every 4–8 weeks; REMICADE 100 mg/vial inj.
10. **Adalimumab:** 40 mg s.c. every 2 weeks; ADFRAR, EXEMPTIA, MABVINTRA 40 mg/0.8 ml inj.
11. **Tocilizumab:** 400 mg infused i.v. over 1 hour every month; TOCIRA, ACTEMRA 400 mg in 20 ml single dose vial.

Note: For preparations of corticosteroids, *see* Index.

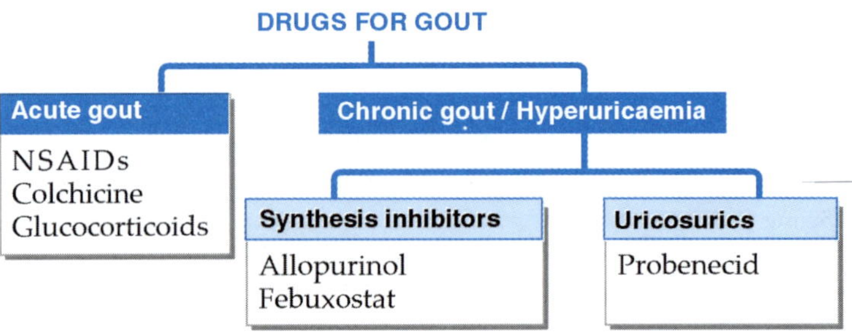

Preparations

1. **Colchicine:** For control of acute attack – 0.5 mg 1–3 hourly to a total of 4 doses in a day, maintenance dose 0.5–1 mg/day; for prophylaxis 0.5–1.5 mg/day; ZYCOLCHIN, GOUTNIL 0.5 mg tab.
2. **Probenecid:** 0.25–0.5 g BD; BENCID 0.5 g tab.
3. **Allopurinol:** Start with 100 mg OD, gradually increase to maintenance dose of 300 mg/day; maximum 600 mg/day. ZYLORIC 100, 300 mg tabs., CIPLORIC 100 mg cap.
4. **Febuxostat:** 40–80 mg OD (max. 120 mg/day). FABULAS, FABUSTAT, ZURIG, FEBURIC 40, 80, 120 mg tabs.

Drugs for Respiratory Disorders

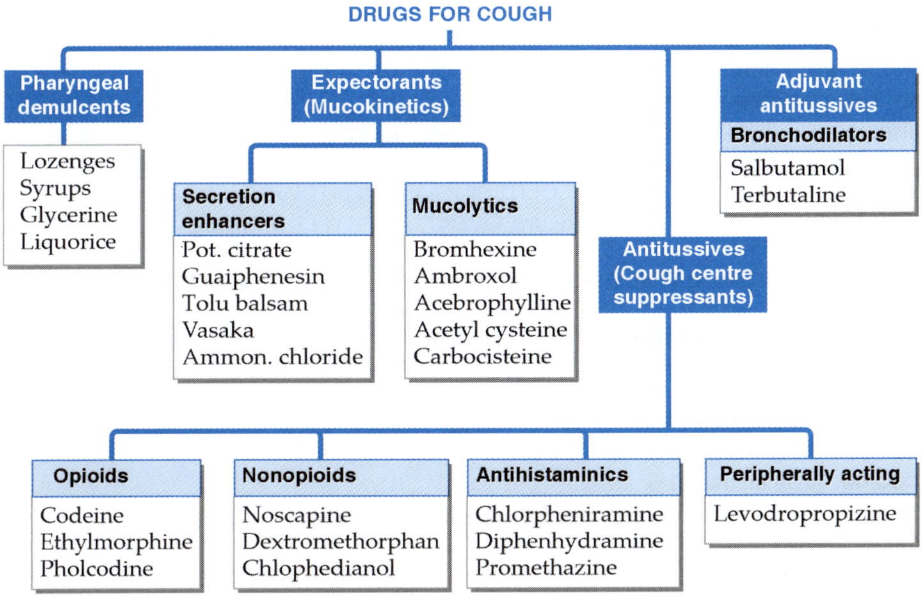

DRUGS FOR COUGH

- **Pharyngeal demulcents**
  - Lozenges
  - Syrups
  - Glycerine
  - Liquorice
- **Expectorants (Mucokinetics)**
  - **Secretion enhancers**
    - Pot. citrate
    - Guaiphenesin
    - Tolu balsam
    - Vasaka
    - Ammon. chloride
  - **Mucolytics**
    - Bromhexine
    - Ambroxol
    - Acebrophylline
    - Acetyl cysteine
    - Carbocisteine
- **Antitussives (Cough centre suppressants)**
  - **Opioids**
    - Codeine
    - Ethylmorphine
    - Pholcodine
  - **Nonopioids**
    - Noscapine
    - Dextromethorphan
    - Chlophedianol
  - **Antihistaminics**
    - Chlorpheniramine
    - Diphenhydramine
    - Promethazine
  - **Peripherally acting**
    - Levodropropizine
- **Adjuvant antitussives**
  - **Bronchodilators**
    - Salbutamol
    - Terbutaline

Preparations

1. Sod./Pot. citrate/acetate: 0.3–1.0 g TDS.
2. Guaiphenesin: 100–200 mg TDS.
3. Tolu balsam: 0.3–0.6 g TDS.
4. Vasaka syrup: 2–4 ml TDS.
5. Ammonium chloride: 50–200 mg TDS.
6. Bromhexine: 8 mg TDS, child 1–5 yr 4 mg BD, 5–10 yr 4 mg TDS; BROMHEXINE 8 mg tab, 4 mg/5 ml elixer.
7. Ambroxol: 30 mg TDS; AMBRIL, AMBROLITE, AMBRODIL, MUCOLITE 30 mg tab, 30 mg/5 ml liq. ACOCONTIN 75 mg CR tab.
8. Acebrophylline: 100 mg 3–4 times a day; ASCOVENT, AB-PHYLLINE 100 mg cap, 200 mg SR tab; 50 mg/5 ml syr., MUCOPHYLLINE 100 mg cap.
9. Carbocisteine: 250–750 mg TDS; in CARBICEF carbocisteine 150 mg + cephalexin 250 or 500 mg caps; BOMOX carbocisteine 150 mg + amoxicillin 250 mg caps.
10. Acetylcysteine: 200–600 mg oral TDS; also by inhalation of 10–20% nebulized solution. FLUIMUCIL 600 mg effervescent tab, MUCOTAB 600 mg tab.; MUCOMIX 200 mg/ml inj in 1, 2, 5 ml amps, PULMOCLEAR acetylcysteine 600 mg + acebrophylline 100 mg film coated tab.
11. Codeine: 15–30 mg TDS; children 2–6 years 7.5 mg, 6–12 years 15 mg.
12. Ethylmorphine: 10-30 mg TDS; DIONINDON 16 mg tab.
13. Pholcodine: 10–15 mg BD–TDS.
14. Noscapine: 15–30 mg, children 2–6 years 7.5 mg, 6–12 years 15 mg; CONOS 25 mg tab, 7 mg/5 ml syr.
15. Dextromethorphan: 10–20 mg TDS, child 2–6 yr 2.5–5 mg, 6–10 yrs 5–10 mg.

16. **Chlophedianol:** 20–40 mg BD–TDS.
17. **Levodropropizine:** 60 mg, children 1 mg/kg 2–3 times a day for not more than 7 days;
    RESWAS levodropropizine 30 mg + chlorpheniramine 2 mg / 5 ml syr.

Some combined antitussive-expectorant formulations

SOLVIN-LS, ASCORIL-LS syrup: Ambroxol 30 mg + Levosalbutamol 1 mg + guaifenesin 50 mg per 5 ml syr.

ASTHALIN PLUS EXPECTORANT: Levosalbutamol 1 mg + guaifenesin 100 mg + ambroxol 30 mg per 10 ml syr.; dose 10–20 ml.

AXALIN EXPECTORANT: Ambroxol 15 mg, guaifenesin 50 mg, terbutaline 1.25 mg per 5 ml syr; dose 5–10 ml.

ZEET syr: Guaifenesin 50 mg, bromhexine 4 mg, diphenhydramine 8 mg, aminon. chloride 100 mg per 5 ml syrup; dose 5–10 ml.

CADICOFF, GRILINCTUS: Dextromethorphan 5 mg, chlorpheniramine 2.5 mg, guaiphenesin 50 mg, Amm. chloride 60 mg per 5 ml syr.

SOLVIN COUGH: Dextromethorphan HBr 10 mg + chlorpheniramine mal. 2 mg per 5 ml syrup.

BENADRYL COUGH FORMULA: Diphenhydramine 14 mg, amm. chlor. 138 mg, sod. citrate 57 mg, menthol 1.1 mg per 5 ml syrup; dose 5–10 ml, children 2.5–5 ml.

BRO-ZEDEX: Bromhexine 8 mg, guaiphenesin 100 mg, terbutaline 2.5 mg, menthol 5 mg per 10 ml syrup; dose 10 ml.

CADISTIN EXPECTORANT: Chlorpheniramine 2 mg, guaiphenesin 80 mg, amm. chlor. 100 mg, sod. citrate 44 mg, menthol 0.8 mg, per 5 ml syrup; dose 10 ml.

CHERICOF: Dextromethorphan 10 mg, chlorpheniramine 2 mg, phenylephrine 5 mg per 5 ml liq.

COSCOPIN LINCTUS: Noscapine 7 mg, chlorpheniramine 2 mg, sod. citrate 3 mg, amm. chlor. 28 mg, per 5 ml syrup; dose 5–10 ml.

GRILINCTUS: Dextromethorphan 5 mg, chlorpheniramine 2.5 mg, guaiphenesin 50 mg, ammon. chlor. 60 mg/5 ml syr; dose 5–10 ml.

M-SOLVIN expecrtorant: Ambroxol 30 mg, guaifenesin 100 mg, terbutalin 2.5 mg tab. and per 10 ml syr.

VENTORLIN EXPECTORANT: Salbutamol 2 mg, guaifenesin 100 mg per 10 ml syrup; dose 10 ml, children 2.5–7.5 ml.

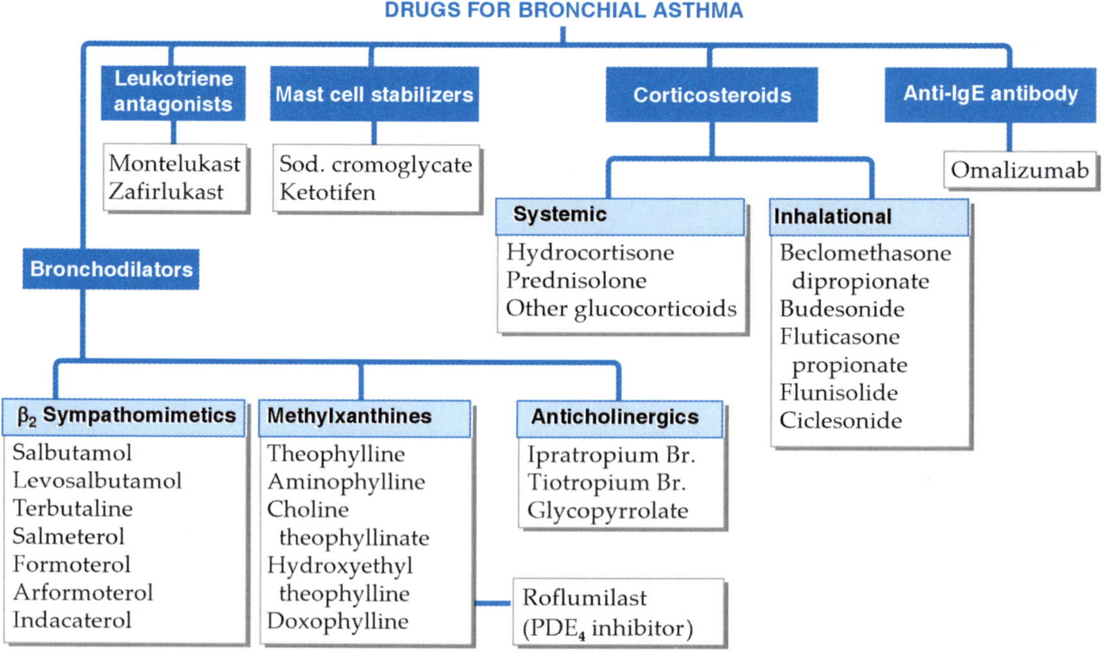
DRUGS FOR BRONCHIAL ASTHMA
Leukotriene antagonists
Montelukast
Zafirlukast
Mast cell stabilizers
Sod. cromoglycate
Ketotifen
Corticosteroids
Systemic
Hydrocortisone
Prednisolone
Other glucocorticoids
Inhalational
Beclomethasone dipropionate
Budesonide
Fluticasone propionate
Flunisolide
Ciclesonide
Anti-IgE antibody
Omalizumab
Bronchodilators
β_2 Sympathomimetics
Salbutamol
Levosalbutamol
Terbutaline
Salmeterol
Formoterol
Arformoterol
Indacaterol
Methylxanthines
Theophylline
Aminophylline
Choline theophyllinate
Hydroxyethyl theophylline
Doxophylline
Anticholinergics
Ipratropium Br.
Tiotropium Br.
Glycopyrrolate
Roflumilast
(PDE_4 inhibitor)

Preparations

1. Salbutamol (Albuterol): 2–4 mg oral, 0.25–0.5 mg i.m./s.c., 100–200 µg by inhalation;
ASTHALIN 2, 4 mg tab., 2 mg/5 ml syrup, 100 µg per puff metered dose inhaler; 5 mg/ml respirator soln., 200 µg rota caps; SALOL 2.5 mg/3 ml inj; VENTORLIN 2 mg/5 ml syr, 4 mg, 8 mg CR caps.
2. Levosalbutamol: LEVOLIN, SALBAIR 50 µg/actuation metered dose inhaler; 0.31 mg (for child 6–11 year) and 0.63 mg (for adult) in 2.5 ml respules for nebulizer; LEVOLIN 1 mg/5 ml syr.; LEVOLIN PLUS: Levosalbutanol + ambroxol 30 mg + guaifenesin 50 mg/5 ml syr.
3. Terbutaline: 5 mg oral, 0.25 mg s.c., 250 µg by inhalation;
BRICAREX 2.5 mg tab.; BRICANYL 0.5 mg/ml inj, 2.5 mg, 5 mg tabs, 1.5 mg/5 ml syr. BRONTALIN 2.5, 5 mg tab.
4. Bambuterol: 10–20 mg oral OD in the evening;
BAMBUDIL 10 mg, 20 mg tabs, 5 mg/5 ml oral soln; BETADAY 10, 20 mg tabs.
5. Salmeterol: 50–100 µg by inhalation;
SALMETER, SEROBID 25 µg per metered dose inhaler; 2 puffs BD; severe cases 4 puffs BD;
SEROFLO—125/250/500 ROTACAPS: Salmeterol 50 µg + fluticasone 125 µg/250 µg/500 µg per rotacap
SEROFLO—125/250, COMBITIDE—125/250, INHALERS: Salmeterol 25 µg + fluticasone 125 µg or 250 µg per puff.
6. Formoterol: 12–24 µg by inhalation twice daily;
FORATEC 12 µg rotacaps. DERIFORM 12 µg/puff metered dose inhaler (MDI). AIRTEC-FF, FORMOSONE: Formoterol 6 µg + fluticasone 125 µg or 250 µg per puff MDI, and respules.
7. Arformoterol: 15 µg by inhalation twice daily; FORATEC 15 µg per puff inhaler, 15 µg/2 ml respules for nebulization.
8. Indacaterol: 150–300 µg once daily by inhalation; ONBREZ 150 µg 300 µg powder filled caps for use in inhaler.
9. Theophylline (anhydrous): 100–300 mg TDS (15 mg/kg/day), THEOLONG 100, 200 mg SR cap., DURALYN-CR 400 mg continuous release cap, UNICONTIN 400 mg, 600 mg CR tabs.

10. **Aminophylline (Theophylline-ethylenediamine; 85% theophylline):** water soluble, can be injected i.v. but not i.m. or s.c., 250–500 mg oral or slow i.v. injection; children 7.5 mg/kg i.v.; AMINOPHYLLINE 100 mg tab, 250 mg/10 ml inj.
11. **Hydroxyethyl theophylline (Etophylline, 80% theophylline):** water soluble; can be injected i.v. and i.m. (but not s.c.), 250 mg oral/i.m./i.v.; DERIPHYLLIN 100 mg tab., 300 mg SR tab., 220 mg/2 ml inj.
12. **Theophylline ethanolate of piperazine:** 250–500 mg oral or i.v.; CADIPHYLLATE, 80 mg/5 ml elixir; ETOPHYLATE 125 mg/5 ml syrup.
13. **Doxophylline:** 400 mg OD-BD, Children 12 mg/kg/day; DOXORIL, DOXOBID, DOXOVENT 400 mg tab, 100 mg/5 ml syr.
14. **Roflumilast:** 500 μg orally once daily; FILAST, ROFLAIR, RUFEN, ROFLU 500 μg tab.
15. **Ipratropium bromide:** 40–80 μg by inhalation; IPRAVENT 20 μg/puff metered dose inhaler, 2 puffs 3–4 times daily; 250 μg/ml respirator soln., 0.4–2 ml nebulized in conjunction with a β_2 agonist 2–4 times daily.
16. **Tiotropium bromide:** 18 μg by inhalation; TIOVA 18 μg rotacaps; 1 rotacap by inhalation OD.
17. **Glycopyrrolate;** 25–50 μg by inhalation once daily; GLYCOHALE inhalation solution as 25 μg respules.
18. **Montelukast:** 10 mg OD; children 2–5 yr 4 mg OD, 6–14 yr 5 mg OD in the evening; EMLUKAST, MONTAIR, VENTAIR 4 mg, 5 mg, 10 mg tabs.
19. **Zafirlukast:** 20 mg BD; children 5–11 yr 10 mg BD; ZUVAIR 10 mg, 20 mg tabs.
20. **Sodium cromoglycate:** 2% by nasal spray (for allergic rhinitis); FINTAL 2% nasal spray.
21. **Ketotifen:** 1–2 mg BD; children 0.5 mg BD; ASTHAFEN 1 mg tab, 1 mg/5 ml syrup; KETASMA 1 mg tab.

22. **Beclomethasone dipropionate:** Initially 100–200 µg BD by inhalation, increase as needed upto 400 µg QID; BECORIDE 50, 100, 250 µg per puff inhaler.
AEROCORT INHALER, SALBAIR-B INHALER 50 µg/metered dose with levosalbutamol 100 µg.
23. **Budesonide:** 200–400 µg BD–QID by inhalation in asthma; 200–400 µg/day by intranasal spray for allergic rhinitis.
BUDECORT: Budesonide 100, 200, 400 µg per puff MDI, 0.25 mg/ml respules.
BUDAMATE INHALER: Budesonide 100 µg/200 µg/400 µg+ formoterol 6 µg per puff MDI.
BUDAMATE TRASCAPS: Budesonide 100 µg/200 µg/400 µg + formoterol 6 µg inhaler caps.
FORACORT: Formoterol 6 µg + Budesonide 100 µg/200 µg rotacaps.
RHINOCORT 50 µg per metered dose nasal spray; BUDENASE AQ 100 µg/metered dose aqueous nasal spray; for prophylaxis and treatment of seasonal and perennial allergic or vasomotor rhinitis, nasal polyposis; initially 2 puffs in each nostril every morning, maintenance 1 puff in each nostril in the morning.
24. **Fluticasone propionate:** 100–250 µg BD (max 1000 µg/day) by inhalation; FLOHALE RESPULES 0.5 mg, 2 mg in 2 ml respules; FLOHALE ROTACAPS 50 µg, 100 µg, 250 µg rotacaps.
FLOMIST 50 µg per actuation nasal spray.
25. **Flunisolide:** 25 µg by local spray in each nostril BD-TDS;
SYNTARIS 25 µg per actuation nasal spray (for allergic rhinitis).
26. **Ciclesonide:** 80–160 µg by inhalation OD in the evening; CICLEZ 80 µg and 160 µg per metered dose inhaler.

Note: For preparations of systemic corticosteroids, *see* Index.

Some combined antiasthma formulations

BRONKOPLUS: Salbutamol 2 mg, anhydrous theophylline 100 mg tab., also per 5 ml syrup.

BRONKOTUS: Bromhexine 8 mg, salbutamol 2 mg tab., also syrup—bromhexine 4 mg, salbutamol 2 mg per 5 ml.

DUOLIN INHALER, COMBIMIST INHALER Salbutamol 100 μg + ipratropium 20 μg per metered dose inhaler.

DUOLIN ROTACAP salbutamol 200 μg + ipratropium 40 μg per rotacap.

DUOLIN RESPULES, COMBIMIST RESPULES salbutamol 2.5 mg + ipratropium 500 μg in 2.5 ml respirator solution.

TERPHYLIN: Terbutaline 2.5 mg, etophylline 100 mg tab and per 5 ml syr.

THEO ASTHALIN: Salbutamol 2 mg, theophylline anhydrous 100 mg tab.

THEO ASTHALIN-SR: Salbutamol 4 mg, theophylline 300 mg SR tab, also syrup—Salbutamol 2 mg, theophylline 100 mg per 10 ml.

THEOBRIC: Terbutaline 2.5 mg, theophylline 100 mg tab.

THEOBRIC SR: Terbutaline 5 mg, theophylline 300 mg SR tab.

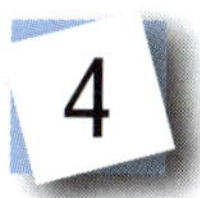

Hormones and Related Drugs

ANTERIOR PITUITARY HORMONES

From acidophil cells

Growth hormone (GH) (Somatropin)
Prolactin

From basophil cells

Thyroid stimulating hormone (TSH)
Adrenocorticotropic hormone (ACTH)
Follicle stimulating hormone (FSH)
Luteinizing hormone (LH)

DRUGS ALTERING ANTERIOR PITUITARY HORMONE SECRETION

Inhibit GH release

Somatostatin
Octreotide
Lanreotide

GH antagonist

Pegvisomant

Inhibit prolactin release

Bromocriptine
Cabergoline

Enhance prolactin release

Chlorpromazine
(other neuroleptics)
Metoclopramide

Inhibit gonadotropin (Gn) release

Superactive GnRH agonists

(Initially enhance Gn release)
Nafarelin, Goserelin
Triptorelin, Leuprolide

GnRH antagonists

Ganirelix
Cetrorelix
Relugolix

Preparations

1. **Growth hormone (Somatropin: recombinant human GH):** For pituitary dwarfism: 0.03–0.06 mg/kg s.c./i.m. in the evening daily or on alternate days. For adult GH deficiency 150–300 μg/day s.c., later adjusted according to response; HUMATROPE 6 mg, 12 mg cartridges, 1.33 and 5.33 mg vials; ZOMACTON 5 mg, 10 mg inj., SAIZEN 5 mg, 8.8 mg inj. EUTROPIN 4 IU inj.
2. **Menotropins (FSH + LH):** obtained from urine of menopausal women: PREGNORM, HUMOG, GYNOGEN 75/150; 75 IU FSH + 75 IU LH activity per amp, also 150 IU FSH + 150 IU LH per amp.
3. **Urofollitropin or Menotropin (pure FSH):** METRODIN, FOLICULIN, SITRODIN HP 75 IU and 150 IU per amp.
4. **Human chorionic gonadotropin (HCG)** derived from urine of pregnant women. CORION, PROFASI, PUBERGEN 1000 IU, 2000 IU, 5000 IU, 10,000 IU, all as dry powder with separate solvent for injection.
5. **Somatostatin:** For upper g.i. bleeding 250 μg slow i.v. injection over 3 min followed by 3 mg i.v. infusion over 12 hours. SOMATOSAN, SOMASTIN 250 μg inj, ZOMATOR 3 mg inj.
6. **Octreotide:** 100 μg i.v. followed by 25 μg/hour; SANDOSTATIN, OCTRIDE 50 μg, 100 μg in 1 ml amp, SANDOSTATIN LAR (microsphere formulation) 10, 20, 30 mg inj.
7. **Bromocriptine:** Start with 1.25 mg BD, titrate upward upto 10 mg BD; PROCTINAL, SICRIPTIN 1.25 mg, 2.5 mg tabs.
8. **Cabergoline:** Start with 0.25 mg twice weekly, increase upto 1 mg twice weekly as needed; CABERLIN 0.25, 0.5 mg tab, CAMFORTE 0.5, 1 mg tabs, CABGOLIN 0.5 mg tabs.
9. **Nafarelin:** For endometriosis 200 μg intranasal spray BD; For precocious puberty 800 μg intranasal spray BD; NASAREL 2 mg/ml solution for nasal spray, 200 μg per actuation.

10. **Triptorelin:** For endometriosis and carcinoma prostate: 3.75–7.5 mg of depot injection i.m. every 4 weeks; For assisted reproduction: 0.1 mg s.c. daily for 10 days starting on 2nd day of menstruation; For precocious puberty: 50 μg/kg i.m. of depot injection every 4 weeks.
    DECAPEPTYL DAILY 0.1 mg inj, DECAPEPTYL DEPOT 3.75 mg inj.
11. **Leuprolide:** For palliative treatment of advanced carcinoma prdostate—1 mg s.c. OD or 3.75 mg i.m./s.c. once a month of depot preparation; LUPRIDE 1 mg inj, 3.75 mg depot inj, LUPRORIN 3.75 mg inj.
12. **Goserelin:** To assist induced ovulation: 3.6 mg depot goserelin i.m. 1–3 weeks before exogenous gonadotropin inj. For endometriosis/carcinoma prostate 3.6 mg every 4 weeks or 10.8 mg every 3 months.
    ZOLADEX 3.6 mg prefilled syringe, ZOLADEX-LA 10.8 mg vial depot injection.
13. **Ganirelix:** 250 μg s.c. in anterior abdominal wall daily from 6th day of cycle, till ovulation is induced
    GANIRELIX ACETATE 250 μg in 0.5 ml prefilled syringe.
14. **Cetrorelix:** 250 μg s.c. daily
    CETROTIDE, CETROLIX 250 μg per vial inj.
15. **Relugolix:** 350 mg oral loading dose on 1st day followed by 120 mg/day.
    ORGOVYX 120 mg tab.

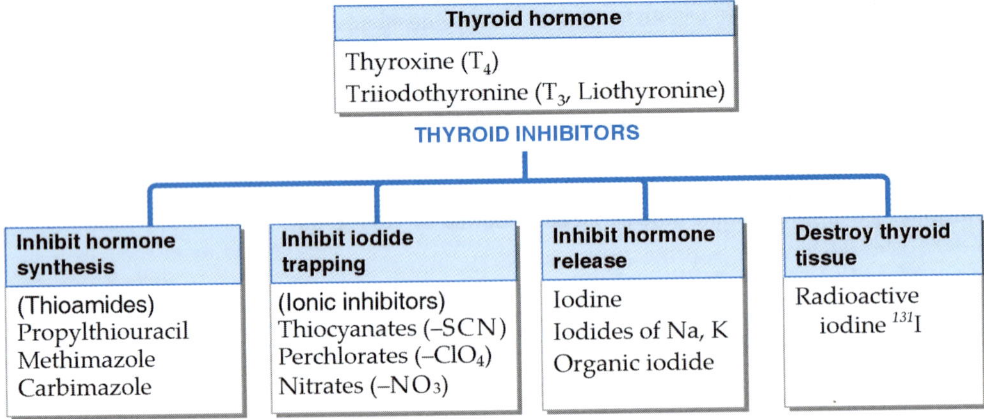
Thyroid hormone
Thyroxine (T_4)
Triiodothyronine (T_3, Liothyronine)
THYROID INHIBITORS
Inhibit hormone synthesis
(Thioamides)
Propylthiouracil
Methimazole
Carbimazole
Inhibit iodide trapping
(Ionic inhibitors)
Thiocyanates (–SCN)
Perchlorates (–ClO_4)
Nitrates (–NO_3)
Inhibit hormone release
Iodine
Iodides of Na, K
Organic iodide
Destroy thyroid tissue
Radioactive iodine ^{131}I

Preparations

L-Thyroxine sod: Adult hypothyroidism—start with 50 μg/day, increase every 2–3 weeks by 25–50 μg to the optimum dose of 100–200 μg/day adjusted by the clinical response and serum TSH level. Cretinism—8–12 μg/kg/day; ELTROXIN, 25, 50, 100 μg tabs, ROXIN 100 μg tab, THYRONORM, 12.5, 25, 50, 62.5, 75, 88, 100, 112, 125, 137, 150 μg tabs, THYROX 25, 50, 75, 100 μg tabs.

1. **Propylthiouracil:** 50–150 mg TDS followed by 25–50 mg BD–TDS for maintenance. PTU 50 mg tab.
2. **Methimazole:** 5–10 mg TDS initially, maintenance dose 5–15 mg daily in 1–2 divided doses.
3. **Carbimazole:** 5–15 mg TDS initially, maintenance dose 2.5–10 mg daily in 1–2 divided doses; NEO MERCAZOLE, THYROZOLE, ANTITHYROX 5, 10, 20 mg tab.
4. **Lugol's solution (5% iodine in 10% Pot. iodide solution):** LUGOL'S SOLUTION, COLLOID IODINE 10%: 5–10 drops/day. COLLOSOL 8 mg iodine/5 ml liq.
5. **Iodide (Sod./Pot.):** 5–10 mg/day prophylactic for endemic goiter; 100–300 mg/day before partial thyroidectomy in Graves' disease.

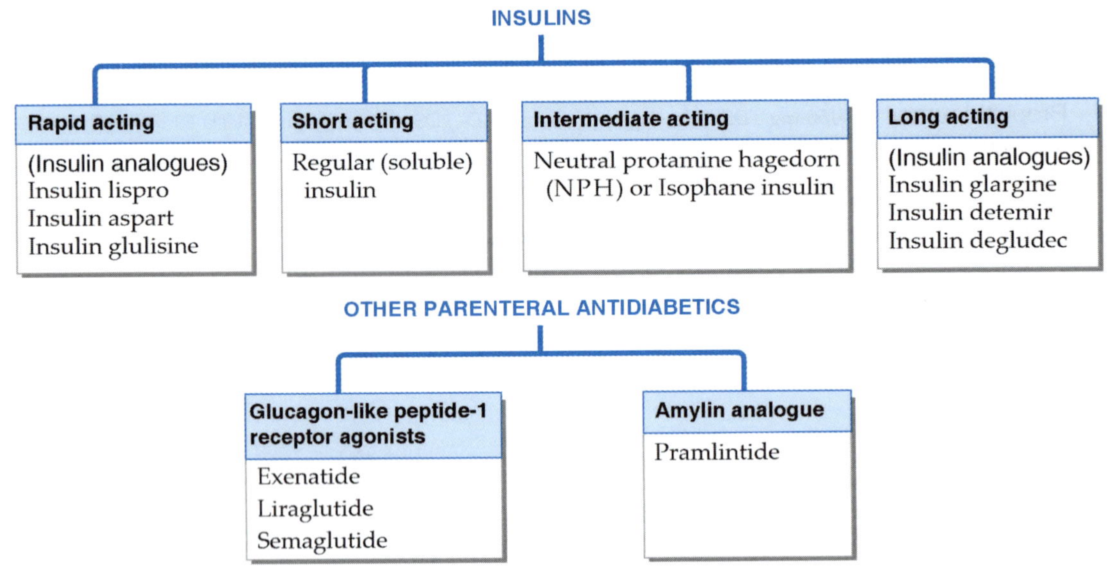
INSULINS
Rapid acting
(Insulin analogues)
Insulin lispro
Insulin aspart
Insulin glulisine
Short acting
Regular (soluble) insulin
Intermediate acting
Neutral protamine hagedorn (NPH) or Isophane insulin
Long acting
(Insulin analogues)
Insulin glargine
Insulin detemir
Insulin degludec
OTHER PARENTERAL ANTIDIABETICS
Glucagon-like peptide-1 receptor agonists
Exenatide
Liraglutide
Semaglutide
Amylin analogue
Pramlintide

Preparations

(Dose to be individualized according to requirement)

1. Human insulins
    1. HUMAN ACTRAPID: Human regular insulin; 40 U/ml, 100 U/ml, ACTRAPID HM PENFIL 100 U/ml pen inj., WOSULIN-R 40 U/ml inj and 100 U/ml pen injector cartridges.
    2. HUMAN INSULATARD, HUMINSULIN-N: Human isophane insulin 40 U/ml, vial and 100 U/ml cartridges for pen injector.
    3. HUMAN ACTRAPHANE, HUMINSULIN 30/70, HUMAN MIXTARD: Human soluble insulin (30%) and isophane insulin (70%), 40 U/ml, and 100 U/ml vial. WOSULIN-30/70 40 U/ml inj and 100 U/ml cartridges.
    4. ACTRAPHANE HM PENFIL: Human soluble insulin 30% + isophane insulin 70% 100 U/ml pen injector.
    5. INSUMAN 50/50: Human soluble insulin 50% + isophane insulin 50% 40 U/ml inj; HUMINSULIN 50:50, HUMAN MIXTARD 50; WOSULIN 50/50 40 U/ml inj. and 100 U/ml cartridges.
2. **Insulin Lispro (rDNA origin):** HUMALOG 100 U/ml, 3 ml cartridge and 10 ml vial and 3 ml Kwikpen; to be injected s.c. within 15 min before or immediately after a meal.
3. **Insulin Aspart:** NOVORAPID, FIASP 100 U/ml inj.
4. **Biphasic insulin aspart:** 70: 30 mixture of isophane insulin aspart with uncomplexed insulin aspart; NOVOMIX 30, FLEXPEN 100 U/ml in 3 ml inj, also as PENFIL injection.
5. **Insulin Glulisine:** APIDRA 100 U/ml in 3 ml cartridge and 10 ml vial, for s.c. inj.
6. **Insulin Glargine:** LANTUS OPTISET 100 U/ml prefilled pen injector.
7. **Insulin Detemir:** LEVEMIR FLEXPEN 100 U/ml in 3 ml pen injector.
8. **Insulin Degludec:** TRESIBA 100 U/ml in 3 ml prefilled flextouch pen, and in 3 ml vial for s.c. inj.
9. **Exenatide:** 5 μg s.c. before breakfast and dinner; 10 mg BD if needed; EXAPRIDE 250 μg/vial inj.
10. **Liraglutide:** 0.6 mg s.c. once daily, increase to 1.2 mg and then 1.8 mg OD if needed. VICTOZA, SAXENDA 1.8 mg/3 ml prefilled syringe delivering 0.6 mg or 1.2 mg or 1.8 mg per dose.
11. **Semaglutide:** 0.25 mg s.c. once a week, increase to 0.5 mg or 1.0 mg per week, if needed.
    OZEMPIC 0.25 mg, 0.5 mg, 1.0 mg single dose prefilled syringe; store at 2-8°C.
    WEGOVY 0.25 mg, 0.5 mg. 1.0 mg, 1.7 mg and 2.4 mg single dose prefilled pens.

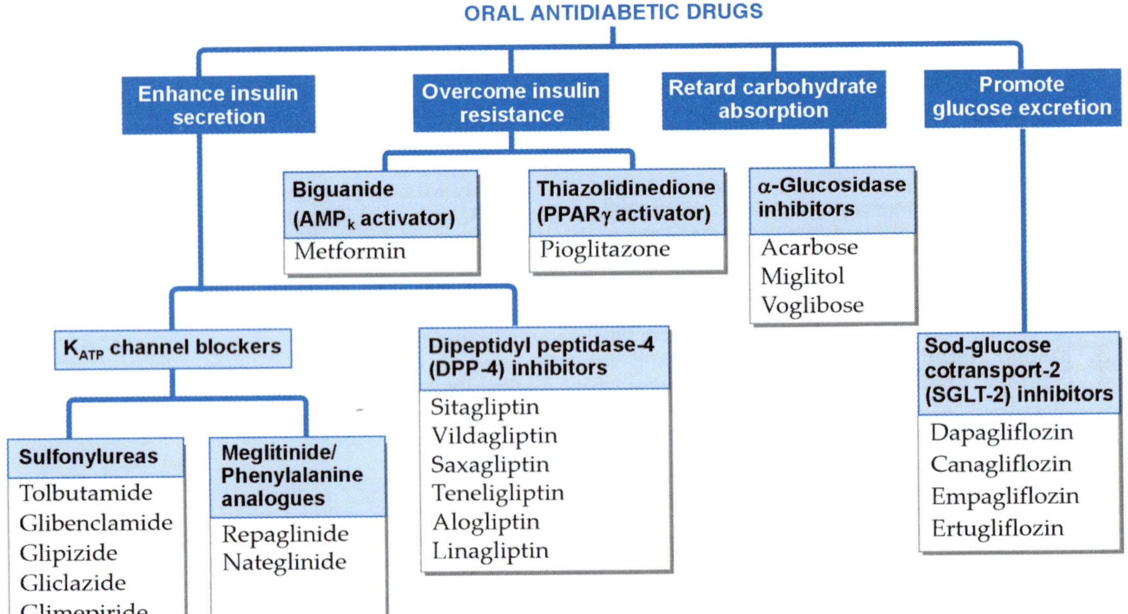
ORAL ANTIDIABETIC DRUGS
Enhance insulin secretion
Overcome insulin resistance
Retard carbohydrate absorption
Promote glucose excretion
Biguanide (AMP$_k$ activator)
Metformin
Thiazolidinedione (PPARγ activator)
Pioglitazone
α-Glucosidase inhibitors
Acarbose
Miglitol
Voglibose
K$_{ATP}$ channel blockers
Dipeptidyl peptidase-4 (DPP-4) inhibitors
Sitagliptin
Vildagliptin
Saxagliptin
Teneligliptin
Alogliptin
Linagliptin
Sod-glucose cotransport-2 (SGLT-2) inhibitors
Dapagliflozin
Canagliflozin
Empagliflozin
Ertugliflozin
Sulfonylureas
Tolbutamide
Glibenclamide
Glipizide
Gliclazide
Glimepiride
Meglitinide/ Phenylalanine analogues
Repaglinide
Nateglinide

Preparations

1. Tolbutamide: 0.5–3 g/day in 2–3 divided doses; RASTINON 0.5 g tab.
2. Glibenclamide (Glyburide): 2.5–15 mg/day in 1–2 doses; DAONIL, EUGLUCON, GLINIL 2.5, 5 mg tab.
3. Glipizide: 5–20 mg/day in 1–2 doses; GLYNASE, GLIDE 5 mg tab.
4. Gliclazide: 40–240 mg/day in 1–2 doses; DIAMICRON 80 mg tab, RECLIDE 30, 60 mg tab, OLIZID 30, 40, 60 mg tabs.
5. Glimepiride: 1–6 mg per day in 1-2 doses; AMARYL, GLYPRIDE, GLMY 1, 2 mg tab.
6. Metformin: 0.5–2.5 g/day in 1–2 doses; GLYCIPHAGE, GLYCOMET 0.5, 0.85 g tab, 1.0 g SR tabs.
7. Repaglinide: 1–8 mg/day in 3–4 doses; EUREPA, PREMEAL, RAPLIN, NOVONORM 0.5, 1, 2 mg tab.
8. Nateglinide: 180–480 mg/day in 3–4 doses; GLINATE, NATELIDE 60, 120 mg tab.
9. Pioglitazone: 15–45 mg OD; PIONORM, PIOREST, PIOZONE 15, 30 mg tab.
10. Acarbose: 50–100 mg TDS taken just before each major meal; GLUCOBAY 25, 50 mg tabs, RECARBS, GLUCAR 25 mg tab.
11. Miglitol: 25-100 mg TDS at beginning of each meal; MIGTOR, DIAMIG, ELITOX 25, 50 mg tab.
12. Voglibose: 0.2-0.3 mg TDS just before meals; VOGLITOR, VOLIX, VOLIBO 0.2 and 0.3 mg tabs.
13. Sitagliptin: 100 mg OD-BD before meals; JANUVIA 50 mg, 100 mg tabs; JANUMET, Sitagliptin 50 mg + metformin 500 mg tabs.
14. Vildagliptin: 50–100 OD or BD before meals; GALVUS, JALRA, ZOMELIS 50 mg tab, GALVUS MET, JALRA-M, ZOMELIS MET: Vildagliptin 50 mg + metformin 500 mg/1000 mg tabs.
15. Saxagliptin: 5 mg OD; half dose in renal failure; ONGLYZA 2.5, 5 mg tabs.
16. Teneligliptin: 20 mg before breakfast daily (max 40 mg/day); TENGLYN, TENEFIT-20, TENLIMAC 20 mg tab.

17. **Dapagliflozin:** 10 mg OD; in liver disease—start with 5 mg OD;
FORXIGA, DAPARYL 5 mg, 10 mg tabs, DAPAGLYL, GLUCRETA 10 mg tab.
18. **Canagliflozin:** 100 mg OD; may increase upto 300 mg OD;
INVOKANA 100 mg, 300 mg tabs; SULISENT, PROMINAD 100 mg tab.
19. **Empagliflozin:** 10 mg OD; may increase upto 25 mg OD;
JARDIANCE, COSPIAO, EMPAONE 10 mg, 25 mg tabs.
20. **Ertugliflozin:** 5 mg OD; may increase upto 15 mg OD;
STEGLATRO 5 mg, 15 mg tabs.

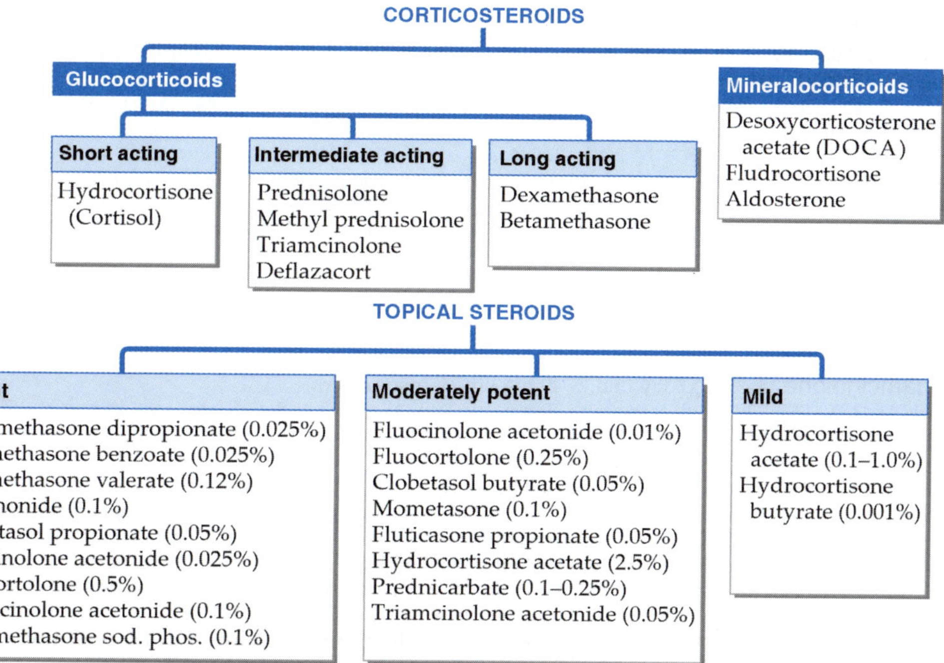
CORTICOSTEROIDS
Glucocorticoids
Mineralocorticoids
Desoxycorticosterone acetate (DOCA)
Fludrocortisone
Aldosterone
Short acting
Hydrocortisone (Cortisol)
Intermediate acting
Prednisolone
Methyl prednisolone
Triamcinolone
Deflazacort
Long acting
Dexamethasone
Betamethasone
TOPICAL STEROIDS
Potent
Beclomethasone dipropionate (0.025%)
Betamethasone benzoate (0.025%)
Betamethasone valerate (0.12%)
Halcinonide (0.1%)
Clobetasol propionate (0.05%)
Fluocinolone acetonide (0.025%)
Fluocortolone (0.5%)
Triamcinolone acetonide (0.1%)
Dexamethasone sod. phos. (0.1%)
Moderately potent
Fluocinolone acetonide (0.01%)
Fluocortolone (0.25%)
Clobetasol butyrate (0.05%)
Mometasone (0.1%)
Fluticasone propionate (0.05%)
Hydrocortisone acetate (2.5%)
Prednicarbate (0.1–0.25%)
Triamcinolone acetonide (0.05%)
Mild
Hydrocortisone acetate (0.1–1.0%)
Hydrocortisone butyrate (0.001%)

Preparations

1. **Hydrocortisone:** 20–30 mg/day oral for replacement therapy; 100 mg i.v. 8 hourly (as hemisuccinate); 100–200 mg i.m./intraarticular (as acetate), 2.0 g as retention enema;
   LYCORTIN-S, EFCORLIN SOLUBLE 100 mg/2 ml vial (as hemisuccinate for i.v. inj.) WYCORT, EFCORLIN 25 mg/ml vial (as acetate for i.m./intraarticualr inj.). PRIMACORT 100, 200, 400 mg/vial inj; HISONE 5 mg, 10 mg tab, 100 mg inj; ENTOFOAM 2 g in 20 g foam cream (10%) for retention enema.
2. **Prednisolone:** 5–60 mg/day oral, 10–40 mg i.m./intraarticular; DELTACORTRIL, HOSTACORTIN-H, 5, 10 mg tab, 20 mg/ml (as acetate) for i.m., intraarticular inj., WYSOLONE 5, 10, 20, 40 mg tab, OMNACORTIL 2.5, 5, 10, 20, 30, 40 mg tabs, 5 mg/5 ml oral susp, 5 mg/ml oral drops. EMSONE 5, 10, 20, 40 mg tab., KIDPRED 5 mg/5 ml syr.
3. **Methyl prednisolone:** 4–32 mg/day oral, 0.5–1.0 g slow i.v. injection for pulse therapy;
   SOLU-MEDROL methylprednisolone (as sod. succinate) 0.5 g (8 ml) and 1.0 g (16 ml) vial, for i.m. or slow i.v. inj., DEESOLONE 4 mg, 16 mg tab, 0.5 g, 1.0 g inj, DEPOT-MEDROL methylprednisolone acetate 40 mg/ml and 80 mg/ml susp for i.m. or intra-articular injection. MEDROL 4, 8, 16 mg tabs.
4. **Triamcinolone:** 4–32 mg/day oral, 5–40 mg i.m./intraarticular;
   KENACORT, TRICORT 1, 4, 8 mg tab., 10 mg/ml, 40 mg/ml (as acetonide) for i.m., intraarticular inj., LEDERCORT 4 mg tab., KENALOG-S EYE 0.1% with neomycin 0.25% and gramicidin 0.025% eye oint., KENACORT, TESS 0.1% triamcinolone acetonide oral paste.
5. **Dexamethasone:** 0.5–5 mg/day oral, 4–20 mg i.v. or i.m.;
   DECADRON, DEXONA 0.5 mg tab, 4 mg/ml (as sod. phosphate) for i.v., i.m. inj, 0.5 mg/ml oral drops; WYMESONE, DECDAN 0.5 mg tab, 4 mg/ml inj, OCUDEX, MINIDEX, DEXONA 0.1% eye drops.
6. **Betamethasone:** 0.5–5 mg/day oral, 4–20 mg i.v./i.m. inj;
   BETNESOL, BETACORTRIL, CELESTONE 0.5 mg, 1 mg tab, 4 mg/ml (as sod. phosphate) for i.v., i.m. inj., 0.5 mg/ml oral drops. BETNELAN 0.5 mg, 1 mg tabs, BETNESOL EYE/EAR 0.1% drops and oint.
7. **Deflazacort:** Initially 60–120 mg/day, maintenance 6–18 mg/day, children 0.25–1.5 mg/kg on alternate days.
   DEFLAR, DEFZA, DFZ 1, 6, 30 mg tabs, DEFGLU 6, 30 mg tabs, DEFCORT 1, 6, 12, 18, 24, 30 mg tabs, 6 mg/5 ml syr.

8. Fludrocortisone: Replacement therapy in Addison's disease 50–200 µg daily. Congenital adrenal hyperplasia in patients with salt wasting 50–200 µg/day. Idiopathic postural hypotension 100–200 µg/day. FLORICORT 100 µg tab.

Topical Steroids

1. Beclomethasone dipropionate 0.025% BECLATE cream
2. Betamethasone benzoate 0.025% TOPICASONE cream, oint.
3. Betamethasone valerate 0.12% BETNOVATE cream, oint., BETASONE cream
4. Halcinonide 0.1% CORTILATE, HALOG cream
5. Clobetasol propionate 0.05% LOBATE, TENOVATE cream
6. Dexamethasone trimethyl-acetate 0.1% MILLICORTENOL cream
7. Fluocinolone acetonide 0.025% FLUCORT oint., LUCI oint.
8. Triamcinolone acetonide 0.1% LEDERCORT oint., KENACORT, TESS buccal paste.
9. Fluocinolone acetonide 0.01% FLUCORT-H oint. and skin lotion
10. Clobetasol butyrate 0.05% EUMOSONE cream
11. Mometasone 0.1% MOMATE, CUTIZONE oint, cream
12. Fluticasone propionate 0.05% FLUTIVATE, MOLIDERM cream
13. Prednicarbate 0.25% DERMATOP, STEROTOP cream
14. Triamcinolone acetonide 0.05% DESONIDE, DESOWEN cream/lotion.
15. Hydrocortisone + (urea 12%) 1% COTARYL-H cream.
16. Hydrocortisone acetate 2.5% WYCORT oint.
17. Hydrocortisone acetate 0.1–1.0% LYCORTIN 1% oint., in CORTOQUINOL 1% with quiniodochlor 4% cream, GENTACYN-HC TOPICAL 1% with gentamicin 0.1%.
18. Hydrocortisone butyrate 0.001% LOCOID cream

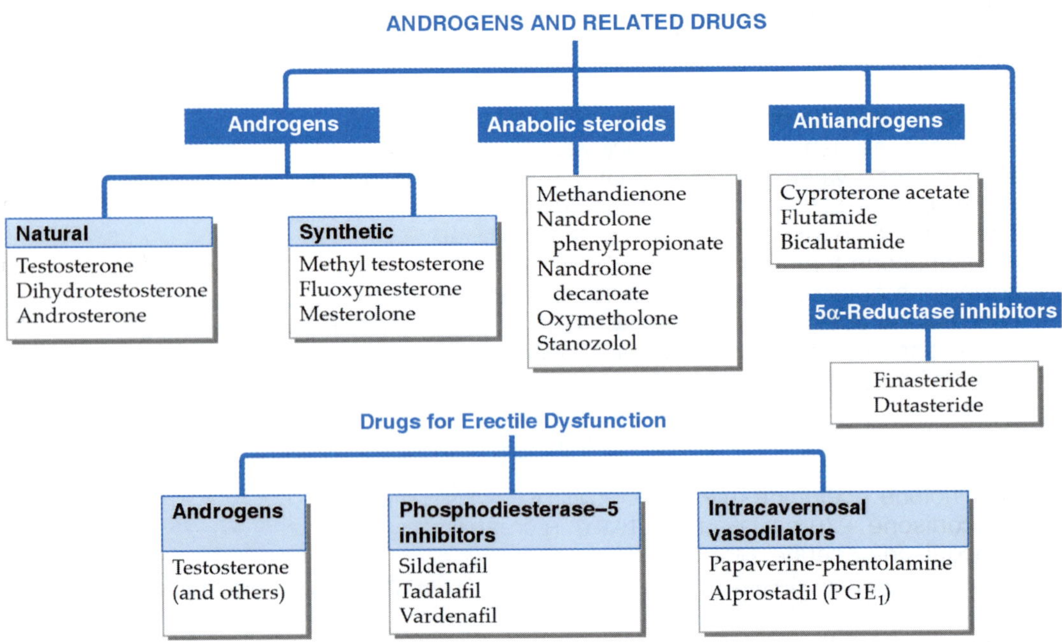
ANDROGENS AND RELATED DRUGS
Androgens
Anabolic steroids
Antiandrogens
Natural
Testosterone
Dihydrotestosterone
Androsterone
Synthetic
Methyl testosterone
Fluoxymesterone
Mesterolone
Methandienone
Nandrolone phenylpropionate
Nandrolone decanoate
Oxymetholone
Stanozolol
Cyproterone acetate
Flutamide
Bicalutamide
5α-Reductase inhibitors
Finasteride
Dutasteride
Drugs for Erectile Dysfunction
Androgens
Testosterone (and others)
Phosphodiesterase–5 inhibitors
Sildenafil
Tadalafil
Vardenafil
Intracavernosal vasodilators
Papaverine-phentolamine
Alprostadil (PGE1)

Preparations

Androgens

1. **Testosterone (free):** 25 mg i.m. daily or twice weekly; AQUAVIRON 25 mg in 1 ml inj.
2. **Testosterone propionate:** 25–50 mg i.m. daily or twice weekly; TESTOVIRON, TESTANON 25, 50 mg/ml inj.
3. TESTOVIRON DEPOT 100: testo. propionate 25 mg + testo. enanthate 100 mg in 1 ml amp; 1 ml i.m. weekly.
4. TESTOVIRON DEPOT 250: testo. propionate 250 mg + testo. enanthate 250 mg in 1 ml amp; 1 ml i.m. every 2–4 weeks.
5. SUSTANON '100': testo. propionate 20 mg + testo. phenyl propionate 40 mg + testo. isocaproate 40 mg in 1 ml amp; 1 ml i.m. every 2–3 weeks.
6. SUSTANON '250': testo. propionate 30 mg + testo. phenylpropionate 60 mg + testo. isocaproate 60 mg + testo. decanoate 100 mg in 1 ml amp; 1 ml i.m. every 3–4 weeks.
7. **Testosterone undecanoate:** NUVIR, AQUAVIRON SOFTGEL, 40 mg cap, 1–3 cap daily for male hypogonadism, osteoporosis.
8. **Mesterolone:** 25 mg OD–TDS oral; PROVIRONUM, RESTORE, MESTILON 25 mg tab.
9. **Testosteron:** 1% gel (transdermal androgen), for once daily application, preferably on upper arm/shoulder; CERNOS GEL, ANDROTAS GEL.

Anabolic Steroids

1. **Methandienone:** 2–10 mg OD oral; children 0.04 mg/kg/day, 25 mg i.m. weekly; DIANABOL 1 mg, 10 mg tabs, DANABOL, DANAMAX 10 mg tab, DANARIX 10 mg/ml amp. for i.m. injection.
2. **Nandrolone phenyl propionate:** 10–100 mg; children 10 mg; i.m. once or weekly; DURABOLIN, NANDROLIN, NANDRIX, ROLONABOL 100 mg/ml inj.

3. **Nandrolone decanoate:** 25–100 mg i.m. every 3 weeks, DECADURABOLIN 25, 50, 100 mg/ml inj.
4. **Oxymetholone:** 5–10 mg, children 0.1 mg/kg, OD; ADROYD 5 mg tab.
5. **Stanozolol:** 2–6 mg/day; MENABOL, NEURABOL, TANZOL 2 mg tab.

Antiandrogens

1. **Cyproterone acetate:** 2 mg OD;
   GINETTE-35, KRIMSON (cyproterone acetate 2 mg + ethinylestradiol 35 μg) tab.
2. **Flutamide:** 250 mg TDS; PROSTAMID, FLUTIDE, CYTOMID 250 mg tab.
3. **Bicalutamide:** 50 mg OD; CALUTIDE, SAMTIDE, TABI 50 mg tab.

5α-Reductase Inhibitor

1. **Finasteride:** For benign hypertrophy of prostate (BHP) 5 mg OD, review after 6 months; for male pattern baldness 1 mg/day. FINCAR, FINARA, FINAST 5 mg tab, FINPECIA, ASTIFINE 1 mg tab.
2. **Dutasteride:** For BHP 0.5 mg/day. DUPROST, DATUS 0.5 mg tab.

Drugs for Erectile Dysfunction

1. **Sildenafil:** 50 mg (max. 100 mg) 1 hour before intercourse; elderly 25 mg;
   PENEGRA, CAVERTA, EDEGRA 25, 50, 100 mg tabs., MANFORCE 50 mg, 100 mg tabs.
2. **Tadalafil:** 10 mg (max. 20 mg) at least ½ hr before intercourse.
   MEGALIS, TADARICH, TADALIS 10, 20 mg tab.
3. **Vardenafil:** 10 mg (elderly 5 mg), max 20 mg ½ to 1 hour before intercourse.
   SAVITRA, VARDITRA, VARDEJUV 5 mg, 10 mg, 20 mg tabs.

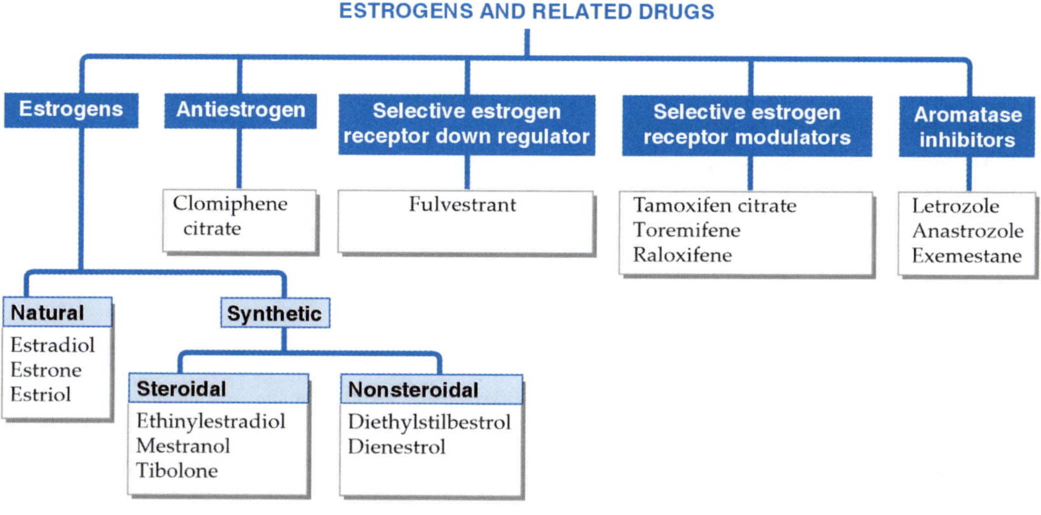
ESTROGENS AND RELATED DRUGS
Estrogens
Antiestrogen
Selective estrogen receptor down regulator
Selective estrogen receptor modulators
Aromatase inhibitors
Clomiphene citrate
Fulvestrant
Tamoxifen citrate
Toremifene
Raloxifene
Letrozole
Anastrozole
Exemestane
Natural
Estradiol
Estrone
Estriol
Synthetic
Steroidal
Ethinylestradiol
Mestranol
Tibolone
Nonsteroidal
Diethylstilbestrol
Dienestrol

Preparations

Estrogens

1. **Estradiol benzoate/cypionate/enanthate/valarate:** 2.5–10 mg i.m.; PROGYNON DEPOT 10 mg/ml inj.
2. **Conjugated estrogens:** 0.625–1.25 mg/day oral for hormone replacement therapy; PREMARIN 0.625 mg, 1.25 mg tab, 25 mg inj (for dysfunctional uterine bleeding). 0.625 mg/g vaginal cream (for atrophic vaginitis) apply 1–3 times per day.
3. **Ethinylestradiol:** for menopausal syndrome 0.02–0.2 mg/day oral; LYNORAL 0.01, 0.05, 1.0 mg tab.
4. **Mestranol:** 0.1–0.2 mg/day oral; in OVULEN 0.1 mg tab, with ethynodiol diacetate 1 mg.
5. **Estriol succinate:** 4–8 mg/day initially, maintenance dose in menopause 1–2 mg/day oral; EVALON 1, 2 mg tab, 1 mg/g cream for vaginal application in atrophic vaginitis 1–3 times daily.
6. **Dienestrol:** 0.01% topical; DIENESTROL 0.01% vaginal cream.
7. **Estradiol transdermal:** ESTRADERM-MX: Estradiol 25, 50 or 100 μg per 24 hr transdermal patches; apply to nonhairy skin below waist, replace every 3–4 days using a different site; add an oral progestin for last 10–12 days every month.
8. **Estradiol dermal gel:** 1–2.5 mg/day; OESTRAGEL, E_2GEL 3 mg/5 g gel in 80 g tube, SANDRENA 1 mg/g gel; apply 1.5–4 g gel over arms & shoulder daily.
9. **Tibolone:** 2.5 mg/day without interruption in postmenopausal women; LIVIAL 2.5 mg tab.

Antiestrogen

Clomiphene citrate: for infertility in women—50 mg/day for 5 days starting from 5th day of cycle, increase to 100 mg/day after 2–3 unsuccessful cycles (max. 200 mg/day); for oligozoospermia in men—25 mg daily for 24 days in a month for upto 6 months; CLOMID, FERTOMID, CLOFERT, CLOME 25, 50, 100 mg tabs.

Selective Estrogen Receptor Down Regulator / Pure Estrogen Antagonist

Fulvestrant: 250 mg (max 500 mg) i.m. (in gluteal region) monthly; FULVENAT 250/vial, and 120 mg/vial inj.

Selective Estrogen Receptor Modulators (SERMs)

1. **Tamoxifen citrate:** 20 mg/day in 1–2 doses (max. 40 mg/day). TAMOXIFEN, MAMOFEN, TAMODEX 10, 20 mg tabs.
2. **Toremifene:** 60 mg OD.
3. **Raloxifene:** 60 mg/day; BONMAX, RALOTAB, ESSERM, RALISTA 60 mg tab.

Aromatase Inhibitors

1. **Letrozole:** 2.5 mg/day oral; FEMARA, ONCOLET, LETOVAL, LETROZ 2.5 mg tab.
2. **Anastrozole:** 1 mg/day oral; ARMOTRAZ, ALTRAZ, ANABREZ 1 mg tab.
3. **Exemestane:** 25 mg/day oral after meals; 50 mg/day in those receiving CYP3A4 inducers; EXMASIN, XTANE 25 mg tab.

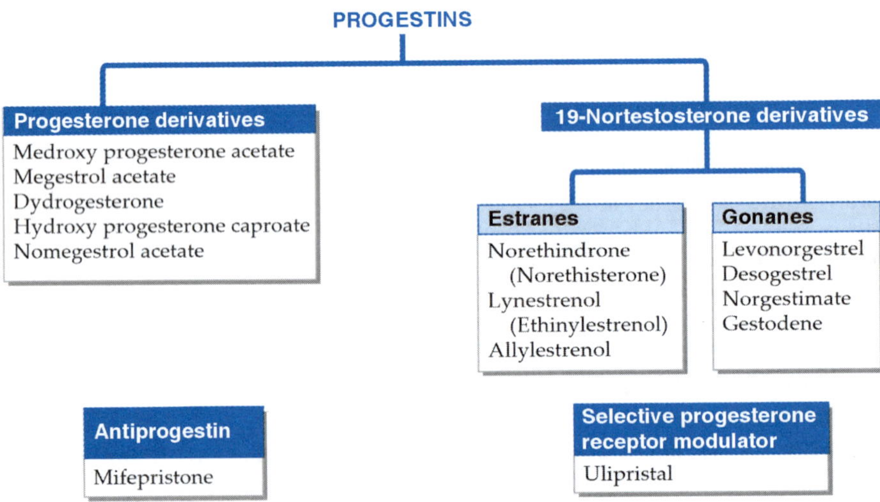
PROGESTINS
Progesterone derivatives
Medroxy progesterone acetate
Megestrol acetate
Dydrogesterone
Hydroxy progesterone caproate
Nomegestrol acetate
19-Nortestosterone derivatives
Estranes
Norethindrone
(Norethisterone)
Lynestrenol
(Ethinylestrenol)
Allylestrenol
Gonanes
Levonorgestrel
Desogestrel
Norgestimate
Gestodene
Antiprogestin
Mifepristone
Selective progesterone receptor modulator
Ulipristal

Preparations

1. **Progesterone:** 10–100 mg i.m. (as oily solution) OD; PROGEST, PROLUTON, GESTONE 50 mg/ml inj., 1 and 2 ml amp; Natural progesterone 100–400 mg OD oral: NATUROGEST, ONGEST, DURAGEST 100, 200, 400 mg caps containing micronized oily suspension. SUSTEN-SR: Natural micronized progesterone 200/300/400 mg SR caps for oral/vaginal administration.
2. **Hydroxyprogesterone caproate:** 250–500 mg i.m. at 2–14 days intervals; PROLUTON DEPOT, MAINTANE INJ 250 mg/ml in 1 and 2 ml amp.
3. **Medroxyprogesterone acetate:** 5–20 mg OD–BD oral, 50–150 mg i.m. at 1–3 month interval; FARLUTAL 2.5, 5, 10 mg tab., PROVERA, MEPRATE 10 mg tab, DEPOT-PROVERA 150 mg in 1 ml inj. (as contraceptive).
4. **Dydrogesterone:** 5–10 mg OD/TDS oral; DUPHASTON 5 mg tab.
5. **Norethindrone (Norethisterone):** 5–10 mg OD–BD oral; PRIMOLUT-N, STYPTIN, REGESTRONE, NORGEST 5 mg tab; REGESTRONE HRT (for HRT); NORISTERAT 200 mg/ml inj (as enanthate) for contraception 1 ml i.m every 2 months.
6. **Lynestrenol (Ethinylestrenol):** 0.5 mg/day as low dose progestin only contraceptive; LYSCOST, WESNOL, DAPHNE 0.5 mg tab.
7. **Allylestrenol:** 10–40 mg/day; GESTANIN, FETUGARD, MAINTANE 5 mg tab, PROFAR 25 mg tab.
8. **Levonorgestrel:** 0.1–0.5 mg/day; DUOLUTON-L, OVRAL 0.25 mg + ethinylestradiol 0.05 mg tab.
9. **Desogestrel:** 150 μg + ethinylestradiol 30 μg (NOVELON) tab, 1 tab OD, 3 weeks on and 1 week off cyclic therapy.
10. **Gestodene:** 75 μg + ethinyl estradiol 30 μg tab; FEMOVAN tab (21 tab pack); MINESSE: gestodene 60 μg+ ethinylestradiol 15 μg tab (24 tab + 4 lactose tab) pack.

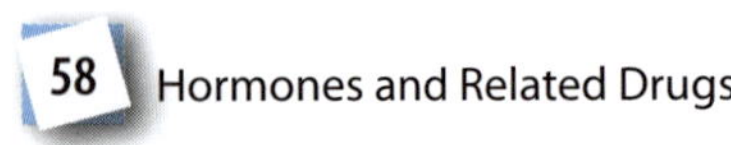

Antiprogestin

Mifepristone: 200–600 mg single oral dose; MIFEGEST, MIFEPRIN 200 mg tab.
MIFEGEST kit, UNWANTED kit: Mifepristone 200 mg 1 tab + Misoprostol 200 μg 4 tabs; take mifepristone 1 tab, followed by 4 tablets of misoprostol orally or inserted intravaginally after 24–48 hours (for abortion within 7 weeks)

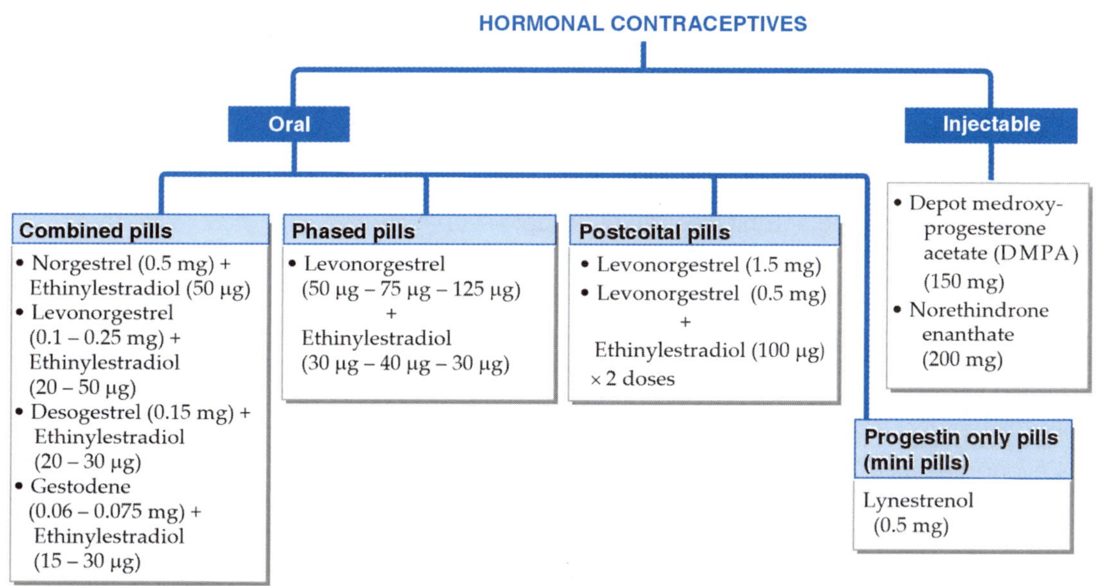
HORMONAL CONTRACEPTIVES
Oral
Injectable
Combined pills
• Norgestrel (0.5 mg) + Ethinylestradiol (50 μg)
• Levonorgestrel (0.1 – 0.25 mg) + Ethinylestradiol (20 – 50 μg)
• Desogestrel (0.15 mg) + Ethinylestradiol (20 – 30 μg)
• Gestodene (0.06 – 0.075 mg) + Ethinylestradiol (15 – 30 μg)
Phased pills
• Levonorgestrel (50 μg – 75 μg – 125 μg) + Ethinylestradiol (30 μg – 40 μg – 30 μg)
Postcoital pills
• Levonorgestrel (1.5 mg)
• Levonorgestrel (0.5 mg) + Ethinylestradiol (100 μg) × 2 doses
Progestin only pills (mini pills)
Lynestrenol (0.5 mg)
• Depot medroxy-progesterone acetate (DMPA) (150 mg)
• Norethindrone enanthate (200 mg)

Combined Pills

1. Norgestrel 0.3 mg + Ethinylestradiol 30 µg: MALAD-D (21 tab.)
2. Norgestrel 0.5 mg + Ethinylestradiol 50 µg; OVRAL-G, 20 tabs.
3. Levonorgestrel 0.25 mg + Ethinylestradiol 50 µg; OVRAL, DUOLUTON-L, 21 tabs.
4. Levonorgestrel 0.15 mg + Ethinylestradiol 30 µg; OVRAL-L, OVIPAUZ, 21 tabs.
5. Levonorgestrel 0.1 mg + Ethinylestradiol 20 µg; LOETTE, OVILOW, COMBEE 21 tabs.
6. Desogestrel 0.15 mg + Ethinylestradiol 30 µg; NOVELON 21 tabs.
7. Desogestrel 0.15 mg + Ethinylestradiol 20 µg; FEMILON 21 tabs.
8. Gestodene 0.075 mg + Ethinylestradiol 30 µg: FEMOVAN 21 tabs.
9. Gestodene 0.06 mg + Ethinmylestradiol 15 µg: MINESSE 24 tabs + 4 lactose tabs.

Phased Pills

1. Levonorgestrel 50–75–125 µg + Ethinylestradiol 30–40–30 µg; TRIQUILAR (6 + 5 + 10 tablets)

Postcoital Pills

1. Levonorgestrel 0.25 mg + Ethinylestradiol 50 µg; OVRAL, DUOLUTON-L (2 + 2 tabs)
2. Levonorgestrel 0.75 mg; ECEE2 (1 + 1 tab)
3. Levonorgestrel 1.5 mg i-PILL, NOFEAR-72, OH GOD (1 tab.).
4. Mifepristone 600 mg; MIFEGEST, MIFEPRIN 200 mg (3 tabs)

Progestin-only (mini) Pills

1. Lynestrenol (0.5 mg): LYSCOST, WESNOL, DAPHNE

Anti-implantation SERM

Centchroman (Ormeloxifene): 30 mg twice weekly for 12 weeks and then 30 mg weekly; CENTRON, SAHELI 30 mg tab.

Injectable Contraceptives

1. **Depot medroxyprogesterone acetate (DMPA):** 150 mg i.m. at 3 month intervals. DEPOT-PROVERA 150 mg in 1 ml vial for deep i.m. injection during first 5 days of menstrual cycle. Repeat every 3 months.
2. **Norethindrone (Norethisterone) enanthate (NEE):** 200 mg i.m. at 2 month intervals. NORISTERAT 200 mg in 1 ml vial for deep i.m. injection during first 5 days of menstrual cycle. Repeat every 2 months.

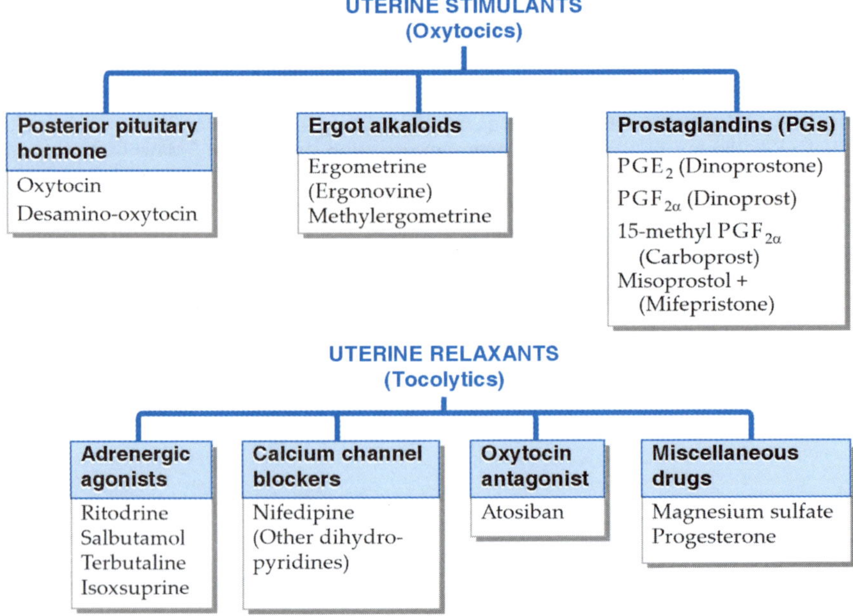
UTERINE STIMULANTS
(Oxytocics)
Posterior pituitary hormone
Oxytocin
Desamino-oxytocin
Ergot alkaloids
Ergometrine
(Ergonovine)
Methylergometrine
Prostaglandins (PGs)
PGE_2 (Dinoprostone)
$PGF_{2\alpha}$ (Dinoprost)
15-methyl $PGF_{2\alpha}$
(Carboprost)
Misoprostol +
(Mifepristone)
UTERINE RELAXANTS
(Tocolytics)
Adrenergic agonists
Ritodrine
Salbutamol
Terbutaline
Isoxsuprine
Calcium channel blockers
Nifedipine
(Other dihydro-
pyridines)
Oxytocin antagonist
Atosiban
Miscellaneous drugs
Magnesium sulfate
Progesterone

Preparations

Uterine Stimulants

1. **Oxytocin:** for induction/augmentation of labour 2–20 milli IU/min i.v. infusion (total 2–4 IU); for postpartum haemorrhage 5 IU i.m. or i.v. infusion;
   OXYTOCIN, SYNTOCINON 2 IU/2 ml and 5 IU/ml inj., PITOCIN 5 IU/0.5 ml inj.
2. **Desamino-oxytocin:** for induction 50 IU buccal every 30 min, for uterine inertia 25 IU buccal every 30 min; for breast engorgement 25–50 IU just before breast feeding; BUCTOCIN 50 IU buccal tab.
3. **Ergometrine:** 0.2–0.5 mg i.m./i.v., 0.25–0.5 mg TDS oral; ERGOMETRINE 0.25, 0.5 mg tab, 0.5 mg/ml inj.
4. **Methylergometrine:** 0.2–0.5 mg i.m./i.v., 0.125–0.25 mg TDS oral
   METHERGIN, METHERONE, ERGOMET 0.125 mg tab, 0.2 mg/ml inj.

Note: For preparations of prostaglandins and uterine relaxants, *see* Index

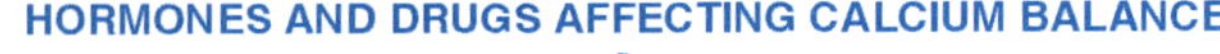

HORMONES AND DRUGS AFFECTING CALCIUM BALANCE

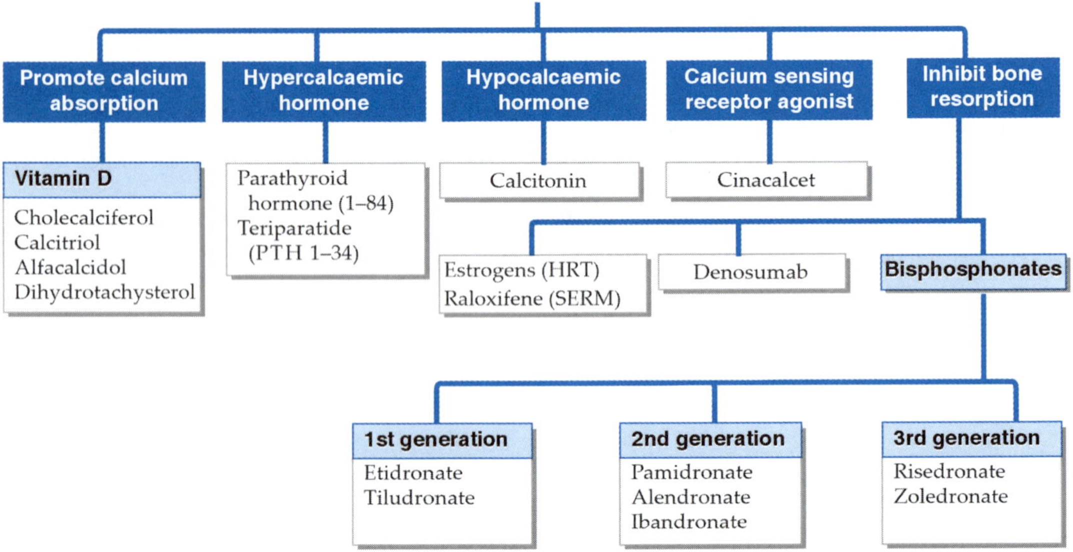

- **Promote calcium absorption**
  - **Vitamin D**
    - Cholecalciferol
    - Calcitriol
    - Alfacalcidol
    - Dihydrotachysterol
- **Hypercalcaemic hormone**
  - Parathyroid hormone (1–84)
  - Teriparatide (PTH 1–34)
- **Hypocalcaemic hormone**
  - Calcitonin
- **Calcium sensing receptor agonist**
  - Cinacalcet
- **Inhibit bone resorption**
  - Estrogens (HRT)
  - Raloxifene (SERM)
  - Denosumab
  - **Bisphosphonates**
    - **1st generation**
      - Etidronate
      - Tiludronate
    - **2nd generation**
      - Pamidronate
      - Alendronate
      - Ibandronate
    - **3rd generation**
      - Risedronate
      - Zoledronate

Preparations

1. Cholecalciferol: CALCIROL, UPRISE-D, ELDECAL-D, LUMIA, CALCIBEST SACHET 60,000 IU in 1 g granules sachet; to be suspended in milk/water and taken at 1–4 week intervals, also soft gel caps and chewable tablets; 1000 IU/5 ml syr, 800 IU/ml drops.ARACHITOL 300,000 IU (7.5 mg) and 600,000 IU (15 mg) per ml oily solution for i.m. injection once a month.
2. Calcitriol: 0.25–1.0 μg orally daily or on alternate days;
   CALTROL, ROLSICAL, ROCALTROL 0.25 μg cap (with calcium carbonate).
3. Alfacalcidol: 1–2 μg/day, children <20 kg body weight 0.5 μg/day;
   ALPHADOL, ONE ALPHA, ALPHA D_3 0.25 μg and 0.5 μg caps.
4. Dihydrotachysterol: 0.25–0.5 mg/day in renal bone disease and hypoparathyroidism.
5. Cinacalcet: 30 mg BD with meals, increase to 60 mg BD or 90 mg BD if needed;
   SETZ 30, 60, 90 mg tabs, PTH-30, SENACEPT 30 mg tab.
6. Teriparatide: 20 μg s.c. once daily;
   TEREOS 750 μg/3 ml vial for inj. TERIFRAC 750 μg/3 ml prefilled cartridge; store at 2-8°C.
7. Calcitonin: For hypercalcaemia: 4–8 μg/kg i.m. every 6–12 hours for not more than 48 hours, or 5–10 IU/kg diluted in 500 ml saline and infused i.v. over 6 hours to supplement bisphosphonates.
   CALSYNAR, ZYCALCIT synthetic salmon calcitonin 100 IU/ml amp. for i.m. or s.c. injection.
   For Pagets disease: 100 IU i.m./s.c. daily or on alternate days for few months.
8. Pamidronate: 60–90 mg infused i.v. over 2–4 hours once a week to once a month;
   BONAPAM, AREDIA, AREDRONATE 30, 60, 90 mg inj.
9. Alendronate: 35–70 mg every week to be taken on empty stomach in the morning with one glass of water. No milk or food to be taken and the subject not to lie down for next 30–60 min;
   OSTEOPHOS, DENFOS 35, 70 mg tabs, RESTOFOS, DRONAL 10, 70 mg tabs.

10. **Ibandronate:** 150 mg once a month orally with the same precaution as for alendronate;
BONIVA, BONRONIC 150 mg tab.
11. **Risedronate:** 35 mg/week or 150 mg/month oral in the morning with precautions as for alendronate;
RISOFOS 35, 75, 150 mg tabs, GEMFOS, ACTONEL 35 mg tab.
12. **Zoledronate:** 4 mg diluted in saline/glucose solution and infused i.v. over 15 min; may be repeated after 7 days and then at 3–4 week intervals;
ZOLDRIA, ZOBONE, ZOLTERO 4 mg/vial inj.
13. **Denosumab:** 60 mg s.c. once every 6 months (for max 3–5 years);
PROLIA 60 mg in 1 ml prefilled syringe (store in fridge).

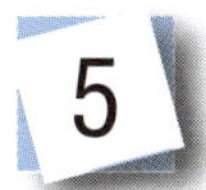

5 Drugs Acting on Peripheral (Somatic) Nervous System

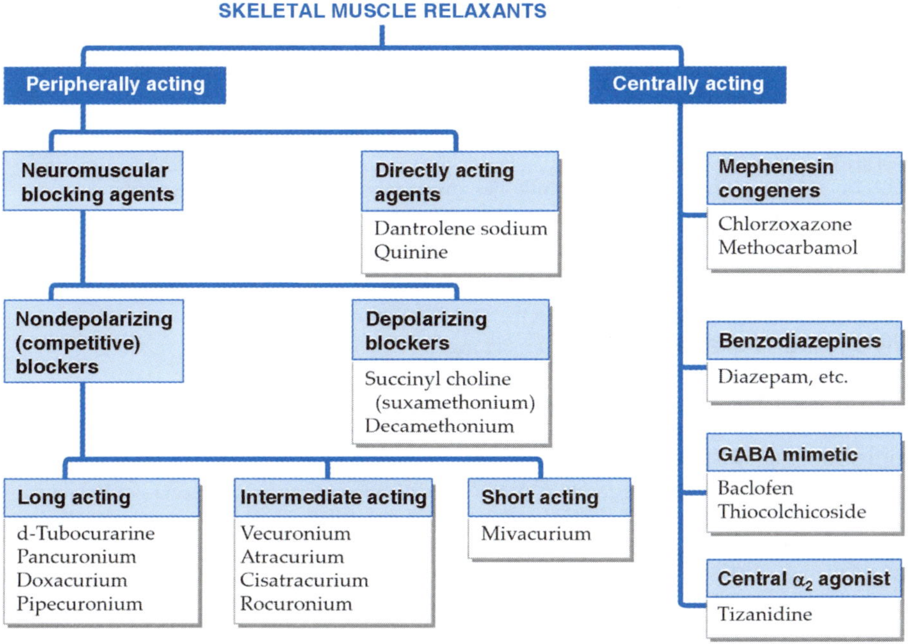

SKELETAL MUSCLE RELAXANTS

- **Peripherally acting**
  - **Neuromuscular blocking agents**
    - **Nondepolarizing (competitive) blockers**
      - **Long acting**: d-Tubocurarine, Pancuronium, Doxacurium, Pipecuronium
      - **Intermediate acting**: Vecuronium, Atracurium, Cisatracurium, Rocuronium
      - **Short acting**: Mivacurium
    - **Depolarizing blockers**: Succinyl choline (suxamethonium), Decamethonium
  - **Directly acting agents**: Dantrolene sodium, Quinine
- **Centrally acting**
  - **Mephenesin congeners**: Chlorzoxazone, Methocarbamol
  - **Benzodiazepines**: Diazepam, etc.
  - **GABA mimetic**: Baclofen, Thiocolchicoside
  - **Central α_2 agonist**: Tizanidine

Preparations

(Note: Doses of neuromuscular blocking agents given below are initial paralysing doses for nitrous oxide-oxygen/opioid anaesthesia. These doses are to be reduced to 1/3 to 1/2 in patients anaesthetised with ether/halothane/isoflurane etc.)

1. Pancuronium: 0.04–0.1 mg/kg i.v.; PAVULON, PANURON, NEOCURON 2 mg/ml in 2 ml amp.
2. Doxacurium: 0.03–0.08 mg/kg i.v.
3. Pipecuronium: 0.05–0.08 mg/kg i.v.; ARDUAN 4 mg/2 ml inj.
4. Vecuronium: 0.08–0.1 mg/kg i.v.;
   NORCURON, NEOVEC 4 mg amp. and 10 mg vial; dissolve in 1–2.5 ml solvent supplied.
5. Atracurium: 0.3–0.6 mg/kg i.v.; TACRIUM 10 mg/ml in 2 ml vial.
6. Cisatracurium: 0.15–0.2 mg/kg i.v.; NIMBEX 2 mg/ml inj.
7. Rocuronium: 0.6–0.9 mg/kg i.v.; ROCUNIUM, ESMERON 50 mg/5 ml, 100 mg/10 ml vials.
8. Mivacurium: 0.15–0.2 mg/kg i.v. MIVACRON 20 mg/10 ml inj.
9. Succinylcholine (Suxamethonium): 0.5–0.8 mg/kg i.v.;
   MIDARINE, SCOLINE, MYORELEX, ENTUBATE 50 mg/ml in 2 ml amp.
10. Dantrolene: 25–100 mg QID oral, 1 mg/kg i.v. repeated as required;
    DANTRIUM 25 mg, 50 mg caps; 20 mg/vial inj., RYANODEX 250 mg/vial inj.
11. Carisoprodol: 350 mg TDS–QID oral; CARISOMA 350 mg tab; SOMAFLAM 175 mg + ibuprofen 400 mg tab.
12. Chlorzoxazone: 500 mg BD–TDS; MOBIZOX 500 mg + diclofenac 50 mg + paracetamol 500 mg tab; PARAFON 250 mg + paracetamol 300 mg tab; FLEXON-MR 250 mg + ibuprofen 400 mg + paracetamol 325 mg tab.
13. Methocarbamol: 400–800 mg TDS oral, 100–200 mg i.m./i.v.;
    ROBINAX 0.5 g tab, 1 TDS: 100 mg/ml inj. for i.v. or i.m. use. ROBINAXOL: methocarbamol 250 mg + paracetamol 350 mg tab.; NEUROMOL-MR 400 mg + paracetamol 500 mg tab.

14. **Baclofen:** 10 mg BD–25 mg TDS oral; LIORESAL, LIOFEN 10, 25 mg tabs.
15. **Thiocolchicoside:** 4–8 mg TDS; NUCOXIA-MR: thiocolchicoside 4 mg + etoricoxib 60 mg tab., THIOCECLO-8, CRITEFEN-T8: thiocolchicoside 8 mg + aceclofenac 100 mg tab.
16. **Tizanidine:** 2 mg TDS; max 24 mg/day; SIRDALUD 2 mg tab; TIZAN 2 mg tab; TREZA 2 mg + ibuprofen 400 mg tab; TIZANAC 2 mg + diclofenac 50 mg tab.

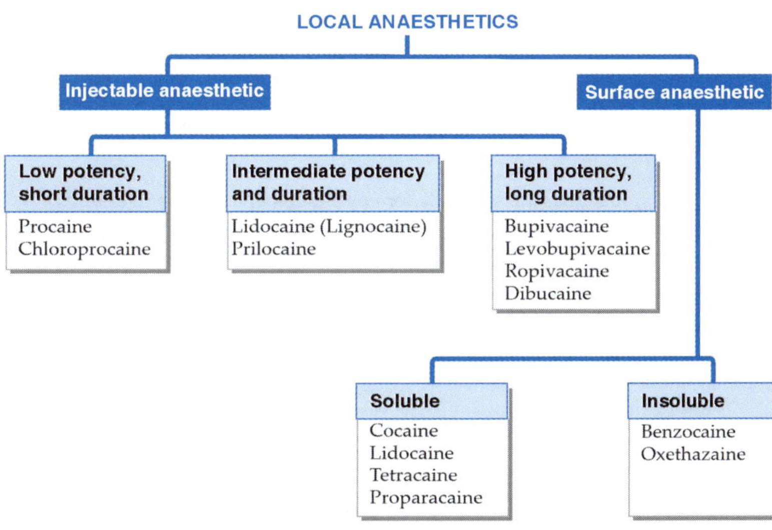

Preparations

1. **Lidocaine (lignocaine):** 0.5–2% for nerve block, 1–5% topically; XYLOCAINE 4% topical solution, 2% jelly, 2% viscous, 5% ointment, 1% and 2% injection (with or without adrenaline), 5% heavy (for spinal anaesthesia); 100 mg/ml spray (10 mg per actuation),
   XYLOCAINE 2% with Adrenaline 1:80,000 in 1.5 ml cartridge for dental anaesthesia.
   PROCTOSEDYL bd: Lidocaine 2.5% + beclomethasone dipropionate 0.025% + phenylephrine 0.1% cream (for application over hemorrhoids)
   LIDOVALOR-EP, DERMALID, LIDODERM 5% patch (for application over bruise, bites, burns, postherpetic neuralgia.
2. **Bupivacaine:** 0.25–0.5% for nerve block, 0.5% for spinal anaesthesia; 0.25–0.5% for epidural anaesthesia, 0.125% for continuous epidural analgesia; MARCAIN 0.5%, also 0.5% hyperbaric for spinal anaesthesia, SENSORCAINE 0.25%, 0.5% inj, 0.5% heavy inj.
3. **Ropivacaine:** 0.75% for spinal anaesthesia, 0.2% for continuous epidural analgesia; ROPIN 0.2% inj.
4. **Eutectic Lidocaine-prilocaine:** 5% for cutaneous anaesthesia; PRILOX, NUMBEX, DOLOCAINE 5% cream.
5. **Proparacaine (proxymetacaine):** 0.5% for ocular anaesthesia; PARACAINE, PROPCAINE 0.5% eye drops.
6. **Dibucaine:** 1% for surface anaesthesia; in OTOGESIC 1% ear drops.
7. **Benzocaine:** 5–20% topically; MUCOPAIN, ZOKEN 20% gel. for mouth ulcers, sore gums etc.
8. **Oxethazaine:** 0.2% for gastric mucosal anaesthesia;
   MUCAINE 0.2% in alumina gel + magnesium hydroxide suspension; 5–10 ml orally.
   TRICAINE-MPS: Oxethazaine 10 mg with methyl polysiloxane 125 mg, alum. hydroxide gel 300 mg, mag. hydroxide 150 mg per 5 ml gel.

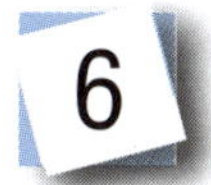

6 Drugs Acting on Central Nervous System

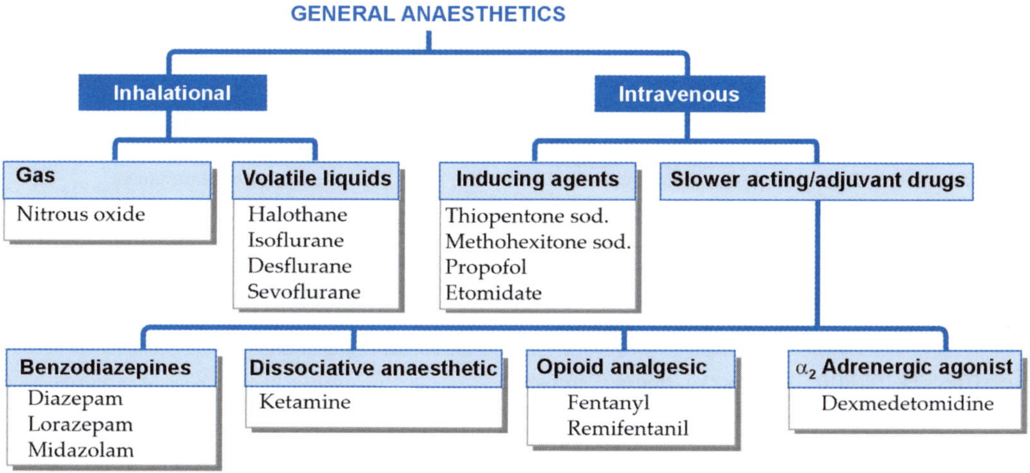

GENERAL ANAESTHETICS

- **Inhalational**
  - **Gas**
    - Nitrous oxide
  - **Volatile liquids**
    - Halothane
    - Isoflurane
    - Desflurane
    - Sevoflurane
- **Intravenous**
  - **Inducing agents**
    - Thiopentone sod.
    - Methohexitone sod.
    - Propofol
    - Etomidate
  - **Slower acting/adjuvant drugs**
    - **Benzodiazepines**
      - Diazepam
      - Lorazepam
      - Midazolam
    - **Dissociative anaesthetic**
      - Ketamine
    - **Opioid analgesic**
      - Fentanyl
      - Remifentanil
    - **α_2 Adrenergic agonist**
      - Dexmedetomidine

Preparations

1. **Thiopentone sod.:** 3–5 mg/kg i.v. for induction;
   PENTOTHAL, INTRAVAL SODIUM 0.5, 1.0 g powder in vial for preparing injectable solution freshly.
2. **Propofol:** 2 mg/kg bolus i.v. injection for induction, 100–200 μg/kg/min for maintenance; 25–50 μg/kg/min for sedating intubated patients.
   PROPOVAN 10 mg/ml and 20 mg/ml in 10, 20 ml vials.
3. **Diazepam:** 0.25–0.5 mg/kg by slow injection in a running i.v. drip; VALIUM, CALMPOSE 10 mg/2 ml inj.
4. **Lorazepam:** 0.04 mg/kg (2–4 mg total for adult) i.v.; CALMESE 4 mg/2 ml inj.
5. **Midazolam:** 1–2.5 mg i.v. bolus injection, 0.02–0.1 mg/kg/hour i.v. infusion for maintenance;
   MEZOLAM, FULSED, SHORTAL 1 mg/ml and 5 mg/ml inj.
6. **Ketamine:** 1–2 mg/kg i.v. or 3–5 mg/kg i.m.;
   KETMIN, KETAMAX, ANEKET 50 mg/ml in 2 ml amp, 10 ml vial.
7. **Fentanyl:** 2–4 μg/kg i.v.; TROFENTYL, FENT, FENDOP 50 μg/ml in 2 ml amp, 10 ml vial.
8. **Remifentanil:** 0.25-0.5 μg/kg/min i.v. infusion;
   REMITHEM 1 mg and 2 mg per vial powder for reconstitution before injection.
9. **Dexmedetomidine:** 0.5–1 μg/kg/hour i.v. infusion;
   DEXDINE, DEXEM, XAMDEX 100 μg/ml inj, 1 ml and 2 ml amp.

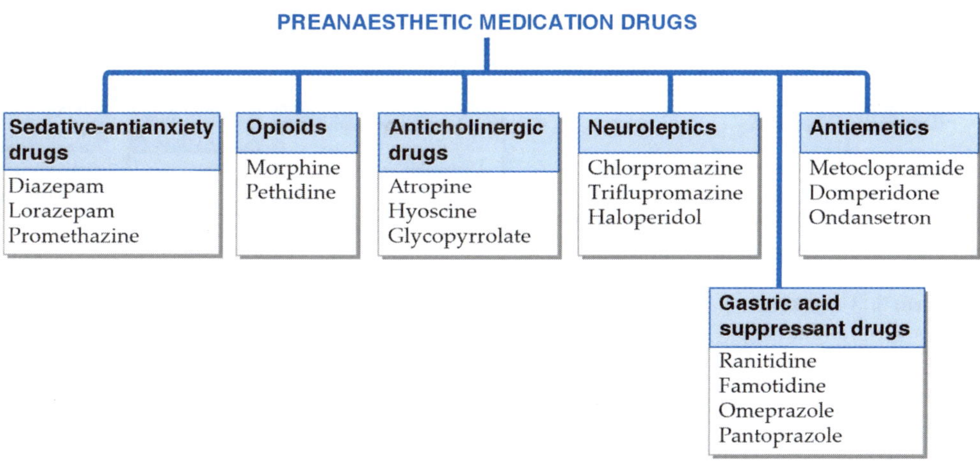

Preanaesthetic Medication Drugs

Note: *See* Index for preparations

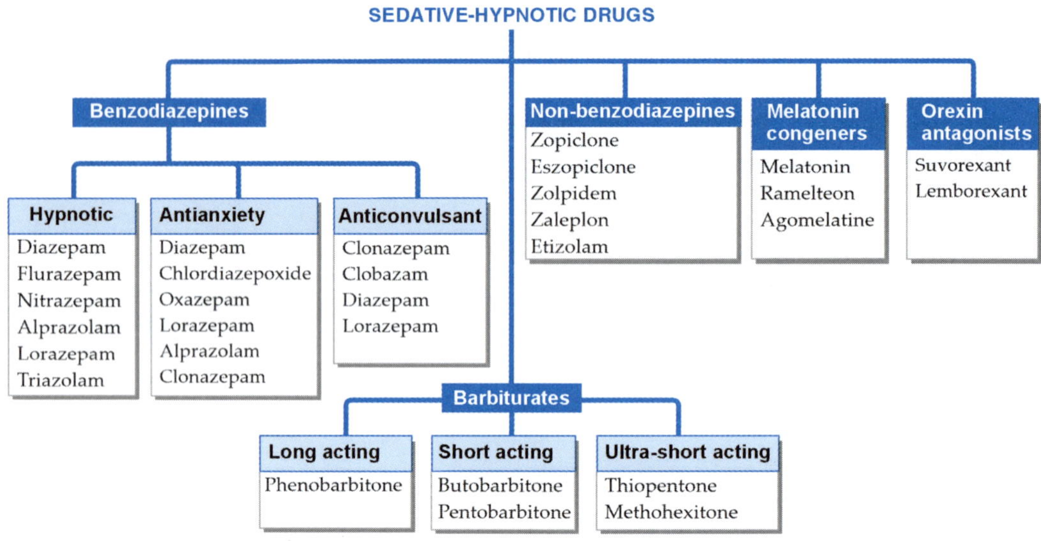

Preparations

1. **Phenobarbitone:** 30–60 mg OD–TDS (as antiepileptic) 100–200 mg i.m./i.v.; GARDENAL 30, 60 mg tab, 20 mg/5 ml syrup; PHENOBARBITONE SOD 200 mg/ml inj.

2. **Diazepam:** 5–10 mg (as hypnotic), 5–30 mg/day (as antianxiety); VALIUM 2, 5, 10 mg tab., 10 mg/2 ml inj., CALMPOSE 5, 10 mg tab, 2 mg/5 ml syr, 10 mg/2 ml inj; PLACIDOX 2, 5, 10 mg tab, 10 mg/2 ml inj.
3. **Flurazepam:** 15–30 mg (as hypnotic); NINDRAL, FLURAZ 15 mg cap.
4. **Nitrazepam:** 5–10 mg (as hypnotic); SEDAMON, HYPNOTEX, NITRAVET 5, 10 mg tab/cap.
5. **Alprazolam:** 0.25–1.0 mg (hypnotic dose), 0.25–1.0 mg TDS for anxiety; ALPRAX 0.25, 0.5, 1.0 mg tabs., 0.5, 1.0, 1.5 mg SR tabs; ALZOLAM 0.25, 0.5, 1.0 mg tabs; 1.5 mg SR tab, RESTYL 0.25, 0.5, 1.0 mg tab, RESTYL-SR 0.5, 1.0, 1.5 mg SR tab, ALPROCONTIN 0.5, 1.0, 1.5 mg CR tabs.
6. **Lorazepam:** 1–2 mg as hypnotic, 1–2 mg 2–3 times a day as anxiolytic; ATIVAN, CALMESE, LARPOSE 1, 2 mg tab.
7. **Triazolam:** 0.125–0.25 mg (as hypnotic).
8. **Zopiclone:** 7.5 mg (hypnotic dose), elderly 3.75 mg; ZOPICON, ZOLIUM, ZOPITRAN 7.5 mg tab.
9. **Eszopiclone:** hypnotic dose 2–3 mg, elderly 1 mg at bed time; FULNITE, ZOLNITE 1, 2 mg tabs.
10. **Zolpidem:** 5–10 mg (max 20 mg) as hypnotic; elderly and liver disease patients 2.5–5 mg; NITREST, ZOLDEM, DEM 5, 10 mg tabs.
11. **Zaleplon:** 5–10 mg (max 20 mg) hypnotic dose; ZAPLON, ZASO, ZALEP 5, 10 mg tabs.
12. **Etizolam:** 1–2 mg at bed time, 0.5–1 mg BD for anxiety; ETIZOLA, ETILAM, ETIREST 0.5, 1.0 mg tabs.
13. **Melatonin:** 3 mg in the evening for jet-lag and disturbed biorhythms; MILOSET 3 mg tab, ZYTONIN, ETERNEX 3 mg + pyridoxine 10 mg tab.
14. **Ramelteon:** 8 mg half hour before bed time; ROZEREM, RAMITAX 8 mg tab.
15. **Agomelatine:** 25–50 mg once at night; AGOPREX, AGOTINE, AGOVIZ 25 mg tab.

16. **Suvorexant:** 10 mg 1/2 hour before going to bed (max 20 mg), elderly 5 mg. BELSOMRA 5, 10, 15, 20 mg tabs.
17. **Lemborexant:** 5 mg before going to bed (max 10 mg); DAYVIGO 5 mg, 10 mg tabs.

Note: See Index for preparations of other drugs.

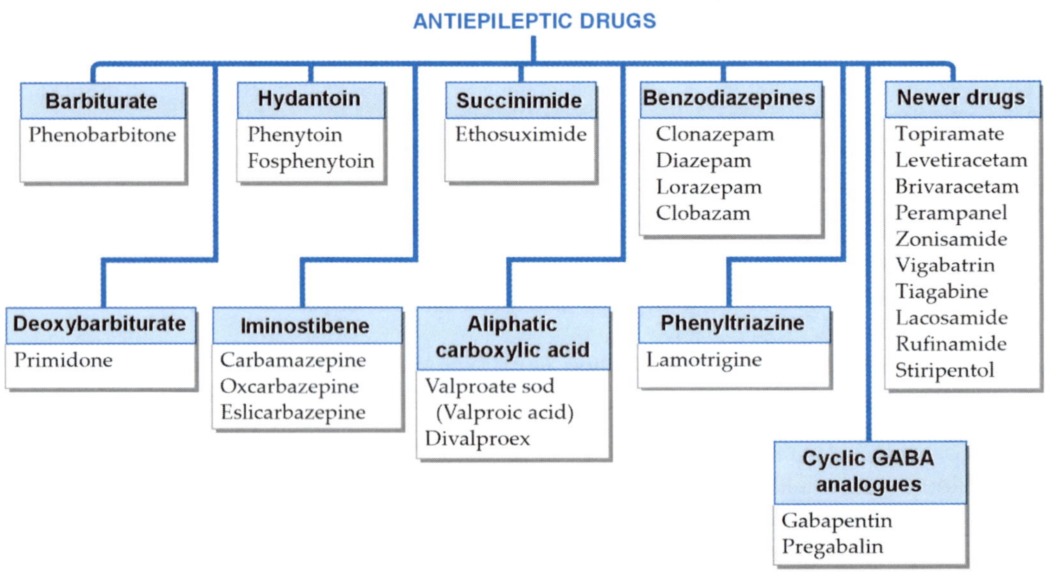

Preparations

1. **Phenobarbitone:** 60 mg OD–TDS (child 3–5 mg/kg/day), 100–200 mg i.m./i.v.; GARDENAL 30, 60 mg tab, 20 mg/5 ml syr.; BARBEE 30, 60 mg tabs.; PHENOBARBITONE SOD 200 mg/ml inj.
2. **Primidone:** 250–500 mg BD (child 10–20 mg/kg/day); MYSOLINE 250 mg tab.
3. **Phenytoin:** 100–200 mg BD (child 5–8 mg/kg/day) oral, 25 mg/min slow i.v. injection (max 1.0 g); DILANTIN 25 mg, 100 mg cap., 100 mg/4 ml oral suspension, 100 mg/2 ml inj.; EPTOIN 50, 100 mg tab., 30 mg/5 ml susp.; FENTOIN-ER 100 mg extended release cap.
4. **Fosphenytoin:** 25-100 mg (as phenytoin sod. equivalent)/min i.v. injection (max 1.0 g) for generalized convulsive status epilepticus; FOSOLIN 50 mg/ml inj in 2 ml and 10 ml amp.
5. **Carbamazepine:** 200–400 mg TDS, children 15–30 mg/kg/day; TEGRETOL, MAZETOL 100, 200, 400 mg tab, 100 mg/5 ml syr; CARBATOL 100, 200, 400 mg tab; MAZETOL-SR, TEGRITAL-CR 200, 400 mg sustained release tabs.
6. **Oxcarbazepine:** 300–600 mg BD; OXCARB, OXEP, OXETOL 150, 300, 600 mg tabs.
7. **Eslicarbazepine:** initially 400 mg/day, increase gradually if needed upto 1200 mg/day; NORMICTAL, ZEFRETOL 400, 800 mg tabs, ESLIFY 200, 400, 600, 800 mg tabs.
8. **Ethosuximide:** 20–30 mg/kg/day; ABSENZ 250 mg/5 ml syr.
9. **Valproic acid (Sodium valproate):** Adults—start with 200 mg TDS, maximum 600 mg TDS; children—15–30 mg/kg/day; VALPARIN CHRONO 200, 300, 500 mg tabs, ENCORATE 200, 300, 500 mg regular tabs and controlled release tabs, 200 mg/5 ml syr, 100 mg/ml inj., VALPROL-CR 200, 300, 500 mg controlled release tabs, 200 mg/5 ml syr, 100 mg/ml inj.
10. **Divalproex:** Epilepsy—initially 15 mg/kg/day, increase gradually as required (max 60 mg/kg/day); Bipolar disorder—250–500 mg TDS; DIPROEX, VALANCE, DEPAKOTE 250, 500 mg tabs.

11. **Clonazepam:** Adults 0.5–5 mg TDS, children 0.02–0.2 mg/kg/day; LONAZEP, CLONAPAX, RIVOTRIL 0.5, 1.0, 2.0 mg tab.
12. **Diazepam:** for status epilepticus—10 mg (0.2–0.3 mg/kg) slow i.v. injection (2 mg/min), repeat fractional doses as required (max 100 mg/day); for febrile convulsions 0.5 mg/kg rectal instillation, repeat 12 hourly for 48 hours; VALIUM, CALMPOSE, PLACIDOX 10 mg/2 ml inj.
13. **Lorazepam:** for status epilepticus—4 mg (0.1 mg/kg in children) slow i.v. injection (2 mg/min); CALMESE 4 mg/2 ml inj.
14. **Clobazam:** start with 10–20 mg at bed time, can be increased upto 40 mg/day; FRISIUM, LOBAZAM, CLOZAM 5, 10, 20 mg cap, CLOBA 2.5 mg/ml susp., CLOBIUM 5 mg/ml susp.
15. **Lamotrigine:** initially 50 mg/day, increase upto 300 mg/day as needed. LAMITOR, LAMETEC, LAMIDUS 25, 50, 100 mg tabs.
16. **Gabapentin:** start with 300 mg OD, increase to 300–600 mg TDS as required; NEURONTIN, GABANTIN 300 mg, 400 mg cap, GABAPIN 100, 300, 400 mg cap.
17. **Pregabalin:** 75–150 mg BD, max. 600/day (used primarily for neuropathic pain). PREGABA, NEUGABA, TRUEGABA 75, 150 mg caps, PREGALIN-X-SR 75 mg SR tab.
18. **Lacosamide:** Start with 50 mg BD, increase upto 200 mg BD as needed; LACASA 50, 100, 150, 200 mg tabs, LACOSAM, LACOPSY 50, 100 mg tabs.
19. **Topiramate:** Initially 25 mg OD, increase weekly upto 100–200 mg BD as required, child 5–10 mg/kg/day. TOPEX, EPITOP, TOPAMATE, NEXTOP 25, 50, 100 mg tabs.
20. **Zonisamide:** 25–100 mg BD (not for children); ZONISEP, ZONICARE, ZONIT 50, 100 mg cap.
21. **Levetiracetam:** 0.5 g BD, increase upto 1.0 g BD; children 4–15 years 10–30 mg/kg/day. TORLEVA, LEVTAM 250, 500, 1000 mg tabs. LEVEPSY, LEVIPIL 250, 500, 750, 1000 mg tabs, 500 mg/5 ml syr, 500 mg/5 ml vial for i.v. injection over 15 min.

22. **Tiagabine:** 4–16 mg TDS; TIGATEL 2, 4, 12, 16 mg tabs.
23. **Brivaracetam:** 25–100 mg twice daily; children 1–2 mg/kg/day in 2 divided doses; BRIVIAPACE, BRIVIACT 50 mg tab, BRIVUP 25 mg, 100 mg tabs., BRITZICAM 25 mg tab.
24. **Perampanel:** Start with 2 mg before bed time, increase upto 8 mg at night; AMPANEL, PERAMPA 4 mg, 6 mg tabs., PERESPY 2 mg, 4 mg tab, HETRAM 2, 4, 6 mg tabs.
25. **Rufinamide:** Children 10 mg/kg/day in 2 divided doses; adults 200–800 mg BD; INOVELON 200 mg, 400 mg tabs.
26. **Stiripentol:** Initially 10 mg/kg/day in divided doses, increase upto 50 mg/kg/day; DIACOMIT 250 mg, 500 mg caps.

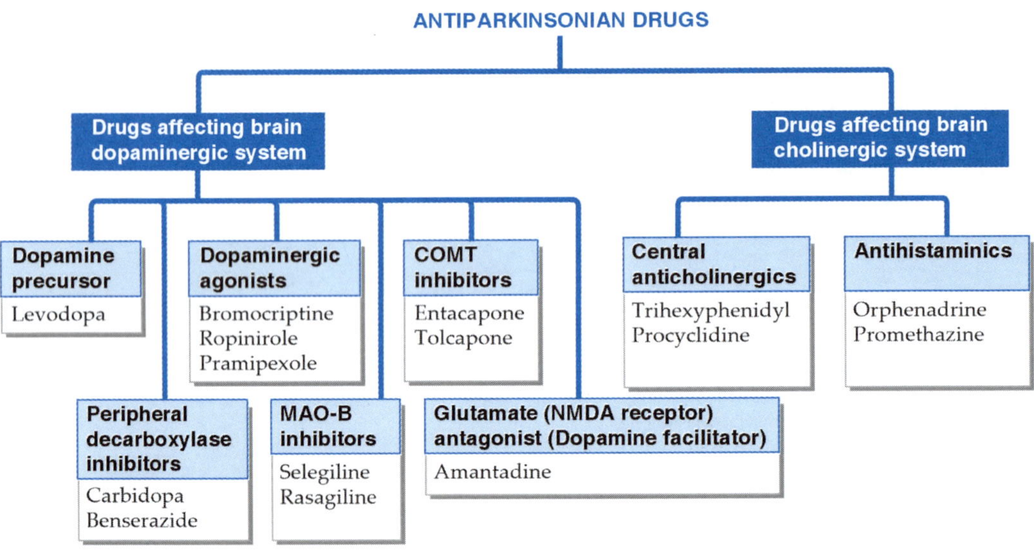
ANTIPARKINSONIAN DRUGS
Drugs affecting brain dopaminergic system
Drugs affecting brain cholinergic system
Dopamine precursor
Levodopa
Dopaminergic agonists
Bromocriptine
Ropinirole
Pramipexole
COMT inhibitors
Entacapone
Tolcapone
Central anticholinergics
Trihexyphenidyl
Procyclidine
Antihistaminics
Orphenadrine
Promethazine
Peripheral decarboxylase inhibitors
Carbidopa
Benserazide
MAO-B inhibitors
Selegiline
Rasagiline
Glutamate (NMDA receptor) antagonist (Dopamine facilitator)
Amantadine

Preparations

1. **Levodopa:** Start with 0.25 g BD after meals, gradually increase till adequate response is obtained. Usual dose is 2–3 g/day. LEVOPA, BIDOPAL 0.5 g tab.
2. **Carbidopa/Benserazide + Levodopa combination:** Usual daily maintenance dose of levodopa is 0.4–0.8 g along with 75–100 mg carbidopa or 100–200 mg benserazide, given in 3–4 divided doses. Therapy is started at a low dose and suitable preparations are chosen according to the needs of individual patients, increasing the dose as required.

	Carbidopa (per tab/cap)		*Levodopa*
TIDOMET-LS, SYNDOPA-110,	10 mg	+	100 mg
SINEMET, DUODOPA-110	10 mg	+	100 mg
TIDOMET PLUS, SYNDOPA PLUS	25 mg	+	100 mg
TIDOMET FORTE, SYNDOPA-275	25 mg	+	250 mg

BENSPAR, MADOPAR: Benserazide 25 mg + levodopa 100 mg cap.

3. **Bromocriptine:** Start with 1.25 mg once at night, increase gradually as needed upto 5 mg TDS, as supplement to carbidopa-levodopa combination.
   PROCTINAL, PARLODEL, SICRIPTIN 1.25 mg, 2.5 mg tabs, ENCRIPT 2.5 mg tab.
4. **Ropinirole:** Starting dose is 0.25 mg TDS, titrated to a maximum of 4–8 mg TDS. Early cases generally require 1–2 mg TDS.
   ROPITOR, ROPARK, ROPIN 0.25, 0.5, 1.0, 2.0 mg tabs.

5. **Pramipexole:** Starting dose 0.125 mg TDS, titrate to 0.5–1.5 mg TDS; PARPEX 0.5, 1.0, 1.5 mg tabs, PRAMIPEX, PRAMIROL 0.125, 0.25, 0.5, 1.0, 1.5 mg tabs.
6. **Selegiline:** 5 mg with breakfast and with lunch, either alone (in early cases) or with levodopa. Reduce by 1/4th levodopa dose after 2–3 days of adding selegiline. ELDEPRYL 5, 10 mg tab, SELERIN, SELGIN 5 mg tab.
7. **Rasagiline:** 1 mg OD in the morning; RELGIN, RASALECT 0.5, 1.0 mg tabs; RASIPAR 1.0 mg tab.
8. **Entacapone:** 200 mg with each dose of levodopa-carbidopa (max 1600 mg/day); ADCAPON, ENTACOM 200 mg tab.
9. **Amantadine:** 100 mg BD. AMANTREL, COMANTREL 100 mg cap.
10. **Trihexyphenidyl (benzhexol):** 2–10 mg/day. PACITANE, PARKIN 2 mg tab.
11. **Procyclidine:** 5–20 mg/day; MODIN 2.5, 5 mg tab.
12. **Orphenadrine:** 100–300 mg/day; ORPHIPAL 50 mg tab.
13. **Promethazine:** 25–75 mg/day; PHENERGAN 10, 25 mg tab.

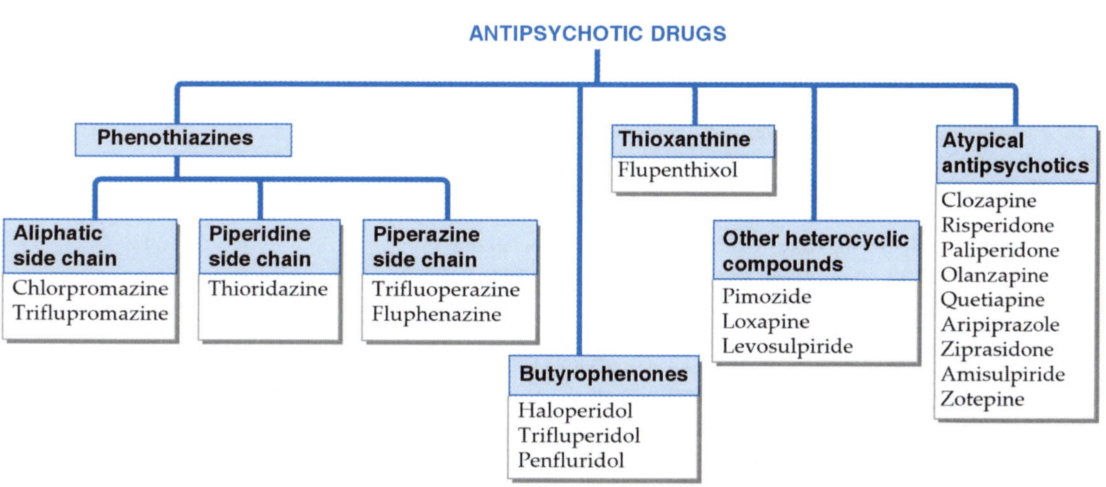
ANTIPSYCHOTIC DRUGS
Phenothiazines
Aliphatic side chain
Chlorpromazine
Triflupromazine
Piperidine side chain
Thioridazine
Piperazine side chain
Trifluoperazine
Fluphenazine
Butyrophenones
Haloperidol
Trifluperidol
Penfluridol
Thioxanthine
Flupenthixol
Other heterocyclic compounds
Pimozide
Loxapine
Levosulpiride
Atypical antipsychotics
Clozapine
Risperidone
Paliperidone
Olanzapine
Quetiapine
Aripiprazole
Ziprasidone
Amisulpiride
Zotepine

Preparations

1. **Chlorpromazine:** 10–100 mg TDS oral/i.m. (max 800 mg/day); CHLORPROMAZINE, LARGACTIL 10, 25, 50, 100 mg tab., 5 mg/5 ml (pediatric) & 25 mg/5 ml (adult) syr., 50 mg/2 ml inj.
2. **Triflupromazine:** 50–200 mg/day; SIQUIL 10 mg tab; 10 mg/ml inj.
3. **Thioridazine:** 25–100 mg 1–3 times a day; MELLERIL 25, 100 mg tab, THIORIL 10, 25, 50 mg tab.
4. **Trifluoperazine:** 2–20 mg/day; TRINICALM 1, 5 mg tab, NEOCALM 5, 10 mg tab.
5. **Fluphenazine decanoate:** 25–50 mg i.m. every 2–4 weeks; ANATENSOL DECANOATE 25 mg/ml for i.m. injection.
6. **Haloperidol:** 2–20 mg/day; SERENACE 1.5, 5, 10 mg tab; 5 mg/ml inj., HALDOL 2, 5, 10, 20 mg tab, 2 mg/ml drops.
7. **Trifluperidol:** 1–8 mg/day; TRIPERIDOL 0.5 mg tab, 2.5 mg/ml inj.
8. **Penfluridol:** 20–60 mg (max. 120 mg) once weekly; SEMAP, FLUMAP, PENRIDOL 20 mg tab.
9. **Flupenthixol:** 3–15 mg/day; FLUANXOL 0.5, 1, 3 mg tab; FLUANXOL DEPOT 20 mg/ml inj. in 1 and 2 ml amp.
10. **Pimozide:** 2–6 mg/day; ORAP, NEURAP, PIMODAC 2, 4 mg tab.
11. **Loxapine:** 10–50 mg BD; LOXAPAC 10, 25, 50 mg caps, 25 mg/ 5 ml liquid.
12. **Levosulpiride:** 25–100 mg 1–3 times a day; LESURIDE 25 mg tab, 75 mg SR tab, 25 mg/2 ml inj, NEXIPRIDE 25, 50, 100 mg tab, 75 mg, 150 mg SR tab, 25 mg/2 ml inj.
13. **Clozapine:** 25–100 mg/day (max 300 mg/day); LOZAPIN, SIZOPIN, SKIZORIL 25, 50, 100 mg tabs.
14. **Risperidone:** 2–8 mg/day; RESPIDON, SIZODON, RISPERDAL 1, 2, 3, 4 mg tabs.
15. **Paliperidone:** Initially 3 mg OD, usual dose 6 mg/day; PALIRIS 3, 6, 9 mg tabs.

16. **Olanzapine:** 5–20 mg/day;
OLACE, OZAP 2.5, 5, 7.5 mg tabs, OLEANZ 2.5, 5, 7.5, 10, 20 mg tabs, 10 mg/amp inj.
17. **Quetiapine:** 50–400 mg/day; QUTIPIN 25, 50, 100, 200 mg tabs, 50, 100, 200, 400 mg SR tabs, SEROQUIN, SOCALM 25, 50, 100, 200 mg tabs.
18. **Aripiprazole:** 10–30 mg/day; ARPIZOL, ARIVE 10, 15, 20, 30 mg tabs., ARILAN 15, 30 mg tabs.
19. **Ziprasidone:** 20–40 mg BD, max 160 mg/day; AZONA, ZIPSYDON 20, 40, 80 mg tabs.
20. **Amisulpiride:** 50–300 mg/day in 2 doses; SULPITAC, SKIZOTUS, AMAZEO 50, 100, 200 mg tabs.
21. **Zotepine:** 25 mg TDS initially, increase upto 100 mg TDS; ZOTIPAX, SIRILEPT 25, 50 mg tabs.

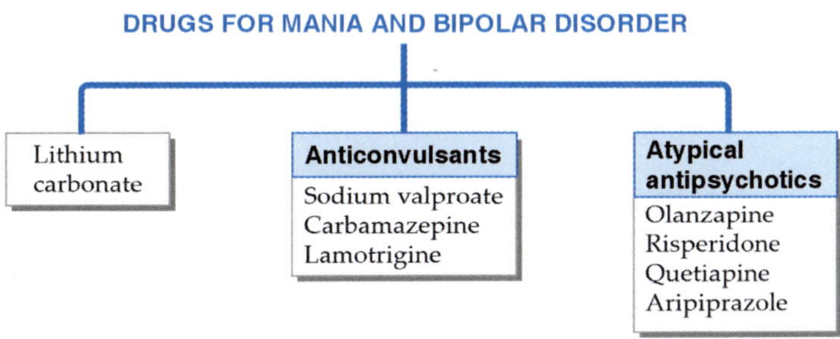

Drugs for Mania and Bipolar Disorder

1. **Lithium carbonate:** Start at 300–600 mg/day, adjust dose to yield steady-state plasma level of 0.5–0.8 mEq/L (for bipolar disorder) or 0.8–1.1 mEq/L (for acute mania);
   LICAB, LITHOSUN 300 mg tab, 400 mg SR tab.

Note: *See* Index for preparations of other drugs.

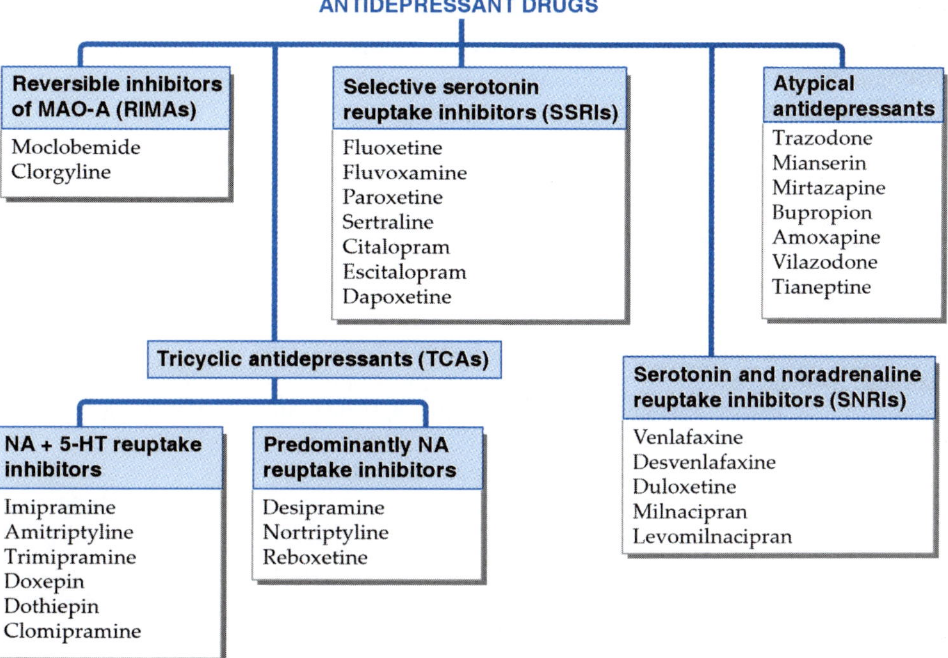
ANTIDEPRESSANT DRUGS
Reversible inhibitors of MAO-A (RIMAs)
Moclobemide
Clorgyline
Selective serotonin reuptake inhibitors (SSRIs)
Fluoxetine
Fluvoxamine
Paroxetine
Sertraline
Citalopram
Escitalopram
Dapoxetine
Atypical antidepressants
Trazodone
Mianserin
Mirtazapine
Bupropion
Amoxapine
Vilazodone
Tianeptine
Tricyclic antidepressants (TCAs)
NA + 5-HT reuptake inhibitors
Imipramine
Amitriptyline
Trimipramine
Doxepin
Dothiepin
Clomipramine
Predominantly NA reuptake inhibitors
Desipramine
Nortriptyline
Reboxetine
Serotonin and noradrenaline reuptake inhibitors (SNRIs)
Venlafaxine
Desvenlafaxine
Duloxetine
Milnacipran
Levomilnacipran

Preparations

1. **Moclobemide:** 150 mg BD–TDS (max. 600 mg/day); RIMAREX, TRIMA 150, 300 mg tabs.
2. **Imipramine:** 50–200 mg/day; DEPSONIL, ANTIDEP 25 mg tab, 75 mg SR cap.
3. **Amitriptyline:** 50–200 mg/day; SAROTENA, TRYPTOMER, 10, 25, 75 mg tabs.
4. **Trimipramine:** 50–150 mg/day; SURMONTIL 10, 25 mg tab.
5. **Doxepin:** 50–150 mg/day; SPECTRA, DOXIN, DOXETAR 10, 25, 75 mg tab/cap; NOCTADERM 5% cream (to relieve itching).
6. **Clomipramine:** 50–150 mg/day; CLOFRANIL 10, 25, 50 mg tab, 75 mg SR tab, CLONIL, ANAFRANIL 10, 25 mg tab.
7. **Dothiepin (Dosulpin):** 50–150 mg/day; PROTHIADEN, EXODEP 25, 50, 75 mg tab.
8. **Nortriptyline:** 50–150 mg/day; SENSIVAL, PRIMOX 25 mg tab.
9. **Reboxetine:** 4–8 mg/day; NAREBOX 4, 8 mg tabs.
10. **Fluoxetine:** 20–40 mg/day; FLUDAC 20 mg cap, 20 mg/5 ml susp; FLUNIL 10, 20 mg caps; FLUPAR, PRODAC 20 mg cap.
11. **Fluvoxamine:** 50–200 mg/day; FLUVOXIN, SOREST 50, 100 mg tab.
12. **Paroxetine:** 20–50 mg/day; XET, PAXIDEP-CR 10, 20, 30, 40 mg tabs.
13. **Sertraline:** 50–150 mg/day; SERENATA, SERLIN, SERTIL 50, 100 mg tabs, ZOSERT 25, 50, 100 mg tabs.
14. **Citalopram:** 20–40 mg/day; CELICA, FELIZ, CITADEP 10, 20, 40 mg tabs.
15. **Escitalopram:** 10–20 mg OD; ESDEP, FELIZ-S, NEXITO 5, 10, 20 mg tabs.
16. **Dapoxetine:** 60 mg 1 hour before intercourse, elderly 30 mg; SUSTINEX, DURALAST, KUTUB 30, 60 mg tabs.
17. **Trazodone:** 50–200 mg/day; TRAZONIL, TRAZALON 25, 50, 100 mg tabs.

18. **Milnacipran:** Initially 25 mg OD, increase every 3 days upto 50 mg BD; MILBORN, MILNACE, MILZA 25, 50 mg caps.
19. **Levomilnacipran:** Start with 20 mg/day, increase upto 120 mg/day; LEVOMIL 20, 40, 80 mg caps.
20. **Amoxapine:** 100–300 mg/day; DEMOLOX 50, 100 mg tab.
21. **Vilazodone:** 20 mg OD after a meal, may increase to 40 mg OD; VILANO, VILAZINE 20 mg, 40 mg tabs., ZOVANE 20 mg tab.
22. **Mianserin:** 30–100 mg/day; TETRADEP 10, 20, 30 mg tab, SERIDAC 10, 30 mg tab.
23. **Bupropion:** 150–300 mg/day; SMOQUIT–SR 150 mg tab.
24. **Mirtazapine:** 15–45 mg/day; MIRT 15, 30, 45 mg tabs, MIRTAZ, MATIZ 15, 30 mg tab.
25. **Venlafaxine:** 75–150 mg/day; VENLOR, SENTOSA 25, 37.5, 75 mg tabs, VENIZ-XR 37.5, 75, 150 mg ER caps.
26. **Desvenlafaxine:** 50–100 mg/day; NEWVEN-OD, VENZ-OD, D-VENIZ 50, 100 mg tabs.
27. **Tianeptine:** 12.5 mg BD–TDS; STABLON 12.5 mg tab.
28. **Duloxetine:** 30–80 mg/day; DELOK, DULANE 20, 30, 40 mg caps, CYMBALTA 20, 30, 60 mg tabs.

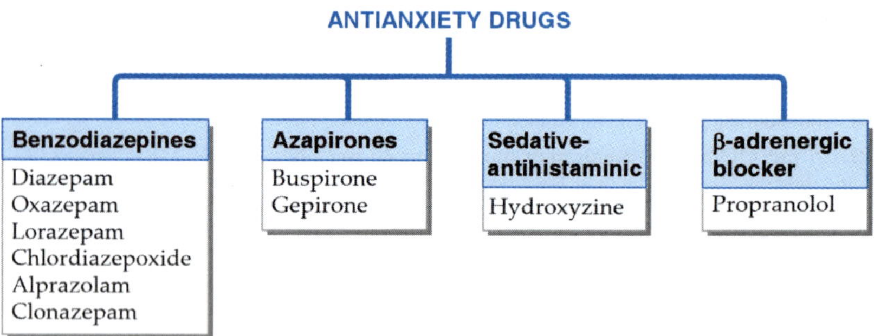

Preparations

1. **Diazepam:** 5–20 mg/day in 2–3 divided doses; VALIUM, PLACIDOX 2, 5, 10 mg tabs; CALMPOSE 5, 10 mg tab, 2 mg/5 ml syr.
2. **Chlordiazepoxide:** 20–100 mg/day in 2–3 divided doses, LIBRIUM 10, 25 mg tabs; EQUILIBRIUM 10 mg tab.
3. **Oxazepam:** 30–60 mg/day in 2–3 divided doses; SEREPAX 15, 30 mg tabs.
4. **Lorazepam:** 1–6 mg/day in 1–2 divided doses; LARPOSE, ATIVAN 1, 2 mg tab. CALMESE 1, 2 mg tabs, 4 mg/2 ml inj.

5. **Alprazolam:** 0.25–1.0 mg TDS; upto 6 mg/day in panic disorder; ALPRAX 0.25, 0.5, 1.0 mg tabs., 0.5, 1.0, 1.5 mg SR tabs; ALZOLAM 0.25, 0.5, 1.0 mg tabs; 1.5 mg SR tab, ALPROCONTIN 0.5, 1.0, 1.5 mg CR tabs. RESTYL-SR 0.5, 1.0, 1.5 mg SR tabs.
6. **Clonazepam:** 0.5–1 mg 1–3 times a day; CLONAPAX, RIVOTRIL, LONAZEP 0.5, 1.0, 2.0 mg tab.
7. **Buspirone:** 5–15 mg 1–3 times daily; BUSCALM, ANXIPAR, BUSPIN 5, 10 mg tabs.
8. **Hydroxyzine:** 50–200 mg/day; ATARAX 10, 25 mg tabs, 10 mg/5 ml syr, 25 mg/2 ml inj.

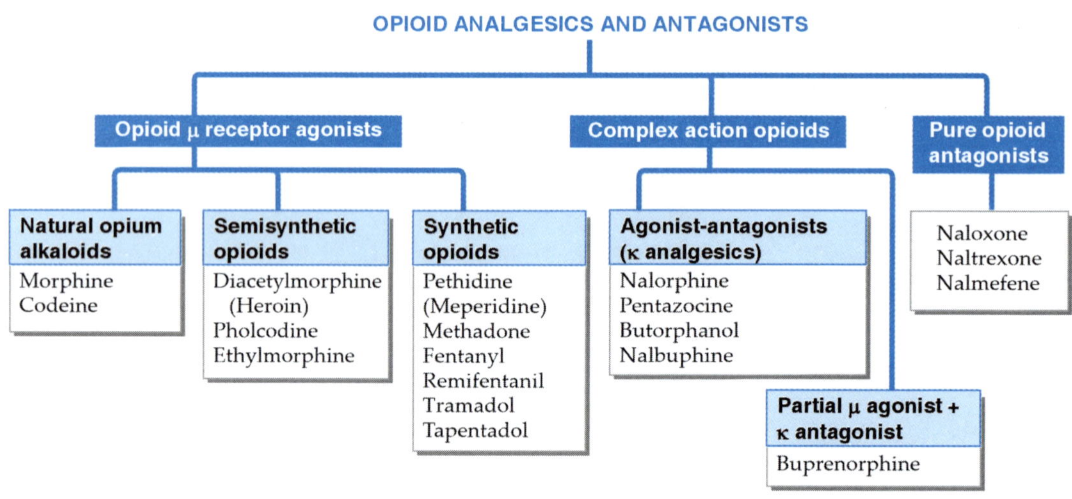
OPIOID ANALGESICS AND ANTAGONISTS
Opioid μ receptor agonists
Complex action opioids
Pure opioid antagonists
Natural opium alkaloids
Morphine
Codeine
Semisynthetic opioids
Diacetylmorphine (Heroin)
Pholcodine
Ethylmorphine
Synthetic opioids
Pethidine (Meperidine)
Methadone
Fentanyl
Remifentanil
Tramadol
Tapentadol
Agonist-antagonists (κ analgesics)
Nalorphine
Pentazocine
Butorphanol
Nalbuphine
Partial μ agonist + κ antagonist
Buprenorphine
Naloxone
Naltrexone
Nalmefene

Preparations

Opioid Analgesics

1. **Morphine:** 10–50 mg oral, 10–15 mg i.m. or s.c., 2–6 mg i.v.; 2–3 mg epidural/intrathecal; children 0.1–0.2 mg/kg i.m. or s.c. MORPHINE SULPHATE 10 mg/ml inj; MORCONTIN 10, 30, 60, 100 mg continuous release tabs; 30–100 mg BD; RUMORF 10, 30 mg tabs., 15 mg/ml inj.
2. **Codeine:** 30–60 mg oral.
3. **Pethidine:** 50–100 mg oral/i.m./s.c., 10–15 mg i.v. (rarely); PETHIDINE 50, 100 mg tabs, 100 mg/2 ml inj, VERPAT 50 mg/ml inj.
4. **Fentanyl:** 2–4 μg/kg i.v.; 12.5–100 μg/hr transdermal; TROFENTYL, FENDOP, FENT 50 μg/ml in 2 ml amp and 10 ml vial, DUROGESIC transdermal patch delivering 12.5 μg/hr, 25 μg/hr, 50 μg/hr, 75 μg/hr and 100 μg per hour; the patch is changed every 3 days.
5. **Remifentanil:** 0.5 μg/kg i.v. injection over 30 sec. followed by 0.25–0.5 μg/kg/min i.v. infusion; REMITHEM 1 mg and 2 mg per vial powder for reconstitution before injection.
6. **Methadone:** As analgesic 2.5–10 mg oral/i.m. (not s.c.); for methadone maintenance therapy 5-40 mg per day.
7. **Tramadol:** 50–100 mg oral/i.m./slow i.v. infusion (children 1–2 mg/kg) 4–6 hourly.
   CONTRAMAL, DOMADOL, TRAMAZAC 50 mg cap, 100 mg SR tab; 50 mg/ml inj in 1 and 2 ml amps.
   ULTRACET, URGENDOL: tramadol 75 mg + paracetamol 325 mg tab.
8. **Tapentadol:** 50–100 mg 2–4 times a day; TAPOSER, DUOVOLT, TAPCYNTA 50, 75, 100 mg tabs; TAPOSER-P: Tapentadol 50 mg + paracetamol 325 mg tab.

Opioid Agonist-Antagonists and Pure Antagonists

1. **Pentazocine:** 50–100 mg, oral, 30–60 mg i.m., s.c., FORTWIN 25 mg tab., 30 mg/ml inj., FORTSTAR 30 mg/ml inj; FORTAGESIC pentazocine 15 mg + paracetamol 500 mg tab.

2. **Butorphanol:** 1–4 mg i.m./i.v.; BUTRUM 1 mg/ml and 2 mg/ml inj.
3. **Nalbuphine:** 10 mg (max 20 mg) i.m./s.c./i.v. every 4–6 hours; NALFY, RUFFY 10 mg in 1 ml and 20 mg in 1 ml inj.
4. **Buprenorphine:** 0.3–0.6 mg i.m., s.c. or slow i.v., also sublingual 0.2–0.4 mg 6–8 hourly; NORPHIN, TIDIGESIC 0.3 mg/ml inj. 1 and 2 ml amps., 0.2 mg sublingual tab; BUPRIGESIC, PENTOREL 0.3 mg/ml inj in 1, 2 ml amp.
5. **Naloxone:** Adults 0.4–0.8 mg i.v. every 2–3 min (max 10 mg); neonates 10 μg/kg in the umbilical cord; NARCOTAN 0.4 mg in 1 ml (adult) and 0.04 mg in 2 ml (infant) amps; NALOX, NEX 0.4 mg inj.
6. **Naltrexone:** 50 mg/day oral; NALTIMA 50 mg tab.

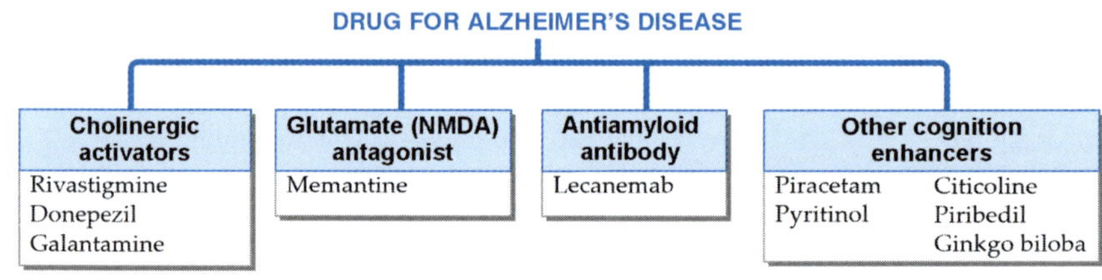

Preparations

1. **Rivastigmine:** Start with 1.5 mg BD, increase every 2 weeks by 1.5 mg/day upto 6 mg/day; EXELON, RIVAMER 1.5, 3.0, 6.0 mg caps.
2. **Donepezil:** 5 mg once at bed time (max. 10 mg OD); DONECEPT, DOPEZIL, DORENT 5, 10 mg tabs.
3. **Galantamine:** 4 mg BD (max. 12 mg BD); GALAMER 4, 8, 12 mg tabs.
4. **Memantine:** 5 mg OD, increase up to 10 mg BD; ADMENTA, MENTADEM 5, 10 mg tabs.
5. **Piracetam:** 0.8–1.6 g TDS; children 20 mg/kg BD–TDS; 1–3 g i.m. 6 hourly in stroke/head injury; NORMABRAIN, NEUROCETAM, NOOTROPIL 400, 800 mg cap, 500 mg/5 ml syr., 300 mg/ml inj.
6. **Pyritinol (Pyrithioxine):** 100–200 mg TDS, child 50–100 mg TDS oral, 200–400 mg 6 hourly (max. 1 g/day) i.v.; ENCEPHABOL 100, 200 mg tab, 100 mg/5 ml susp, 200 mg dry powder in vial with solvent for i.v. infusion.
7. **Piribedil:** 50 mg OD–BD; TRIVASTAL-LA 50 mg tab.
8. **Ginkgo biloba:** 40–80 mg TDS; GINKOCER, BILOVAS, GINKOBA 40 mg tab.
9. **Citicoline:** 500 mg OD-BD (max 2 g/day) oral; 0.5–1.0 g/day i.v. or i.m. STROLIN 500 mg tab, CITILINE, CITINOVA 500 mg tab, 500 mg/2 ml inj.

7 Cardiovascular Drugs

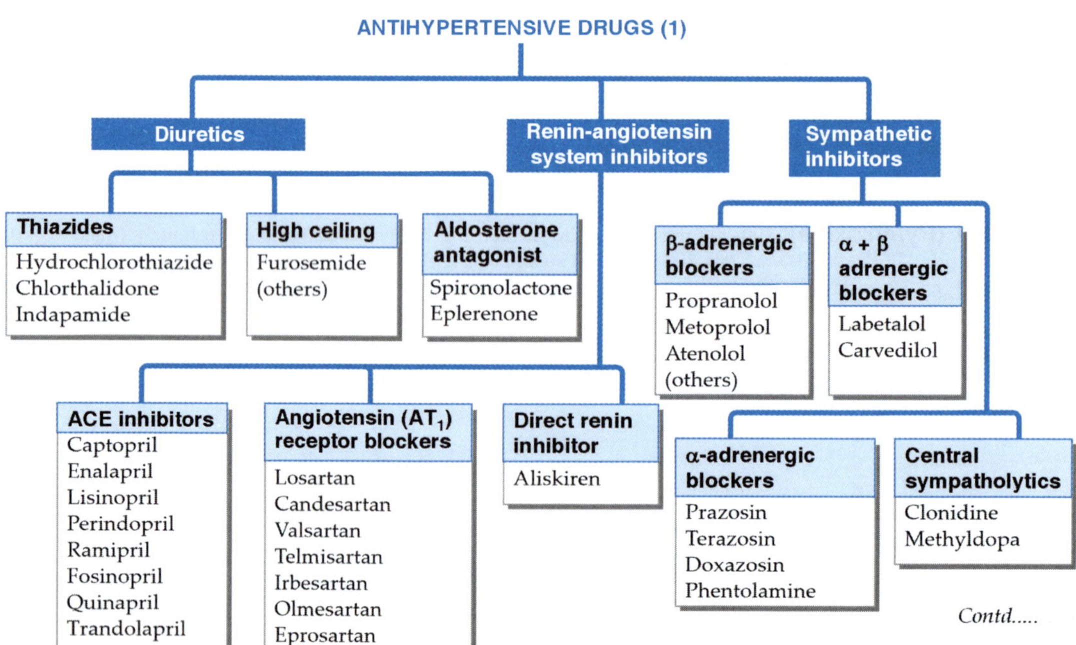

Contd.....

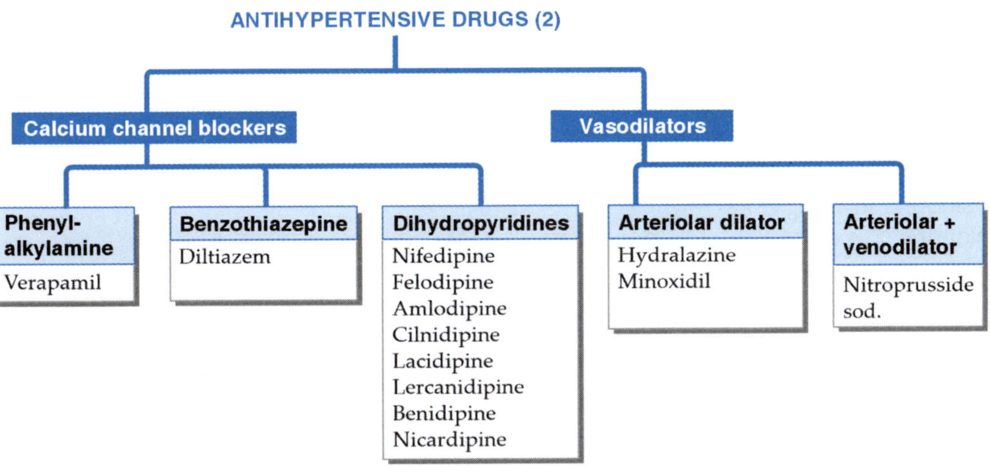
ANTIHYPERTENSIVE DRUGS (2)
Calcium channel blockers
Vasodilators
Phenyl-alkylamine
Verapamil
Benzothiazepine
Diltiazem
Dihydropyridines
Nifedipine
Felodipine
Amlodipine
Cilnidipine
Lacidipine
Lercanidipine
Benidipine
Nicardipine
Arteriolar dilator
Hydralazine
Minoxidil
Arteriolar + venodilator
Nitroprusside sod.

Preparations

1. **Captopril:** Initially 25 mg BD, increase upto 50 mg TDS as needed. To be taken 1 hr before or 2 hr after a meal; ANGIOPRIL 25 mg tab, ACETEN, 12.5, 25 mg tabs.
2. **Enalapril:** 2.5 mg OD–20 mg BD; ENAPRIL, ENVAS, ENAM 2.5, 5, 10, 20 mg tabs.
3. **Lisinopril:** 5 mg OD–20 mg BD; LINVAS, LISTRIL, LIPRIL 2.5, 5, 10 mg tabs, LISORIL 2.5, 5, 10, 20 mg tabs.
4. **Perindopril:** 2 mg OD–4 mg BD; COVERSYL 2, 4 mg tabs.
5. **Ramipril:** 1.25 mg OD–5 mg BD; CARDACE, RAMIRIL, CORPRIL, R.PRIL 1.25, 2.5, 5 mg caps.
6. **Benazepril:** 10 mg OD–20 mg BD; BENACE 5, 10, 20 mg tabs.
7. **Trandolapril:** 2 mg OD–4 mg BD; ZETPRIL 1, 2 mg tabs.
8. **Fosinopril:** 10–40 mg OD; FOSINACE, FOVAS 10, 20 mg tabs.
9. **Imidapril:** Start with 5 mg (elderly 2.5 mg) OD, max. 10 mg OD; TANATRIL 5, 10 mg tabs.
10. **Quinapril:** 10–40 mg/day; Q-PRESS-H Quinapril 20 mg + hydrochlorothiazide 12.5 mg tab.
11. **Losartan:** 50 mg OD (max. 50 mg BD), liver disease and volume depleted patients 25 mg OD; LOSAR, LOSACAR, TOZAAR, ALSARTAN 25, 50 mg tabs.
12. **Candesartan:** 8 mg OD (max. 8 mg BD), liver/kidney disease patients 4 mg OD; CANDESAR, CANDILONG, CANDESTAN 4, 8 mg tabs.
13. **Irbesartan:** 150–300 mg OD; IROVEL, IRBEST 150, 300 mg tabs.
14. **Valsartan:** 80–160 mg OD; DIOVAN 40, 80, 160 mg tabs. STARVAL, VALZAAR 80, 160 mg tabs.
15. **Telmisartan:** 20–80 mg OD; TELMA, TELSAR, TELVAS 20, 40, 80 mg tabs.
16. **Olmesartan medoxomil:** 20–40 mg OD; OLMAT, OLSAR 20, 40 mg tabs.
17. **Eprosartan:** 600 mg OD; EPROZAR 600 mg tab.

18. **Aliskiren:** 150–300 mg OD; RASILEZ 150 mg tab; RASILEZ-HC alongwith hydrochlorothiazide 12.5 mg.
19. **Verapamil:** 40–160 mg TDS oral, 5 mg by slow i.v. inj; CALAPTIN 40, 80 mg tab, 120, 240 mg SR tab; 5 mg/2 ml inj, VASOPTEN 40, 80, 120 mg tabs.
20. **Diltiazem:** 30–60 mg TDS–QID oral; DILZEM 30, 60 mg tabs, 90 mg SR tab; 25 mg/5 ml inj; ANGIZEM 30, 60, 90, 120, 180 mg tab, DILTIME 30, 60 mg tab; 90, 120 mg SR tab.
21. **Nifedipine:** 5–20 mg BD–TDS oral; CALCIGARD, DEPIN, NIFELAT 5, 10 mg cap, also 10 mg, 20 mg SR (RETARD) tab., ADALAT RETARD 10, 20 mg SR tab.
22. **Felodipine:** 5–10 mg OD (max. 10 mg BD); FELOGARD, PLENDIL, RENDIL 2.5, 5, 10 mg ER tab.
23. **Amlodipine:** 5–10 mg OD; AMLOPRES, AMCARD, AMLOPIN, MYODURA 2.5, 5, 10 mg tabs.
24. **S(–) Amlodipine:** 2.5–5 mg OD; S-NUMLO 1.25, 2.5, 5.0 mg tabs; S-AMCARD, ASOMEX 2.5, 5.0 mg tabs.
25. **Nitrendipine:** 5–20 mg OD; CARDIF, NITREPIN 10, 20 mg tab.
26. **Cilnidipine:** 5–20 mg OD; CILACAR, CILAGARD 5, 10 mg tab.
27. **Lacidipine:** 4–6 mg OD; LACIVAS, SINOPIL 2, 4 mg tabs.
28. **Benidipine:** 4–8 mg OD; CARITEC 4, 8 mg tabs.
29. **Lercanidipine:** 10–20 mg OD; LERKA 10, 20 mg tabs.
30. **Nicardipine:** 20–40 mg TDS oral, 30–60 mg BD as ER tab; 5–15 mg/hr i.v. infusion; NICARDIPINE 25 mg/10 ml inj.
31. **Hydrochlorothiazide:** 12.5–50 mg OD; AQUAZIDE. THIAZIDE, HYDRIDE 12.5, 25, 50 mg tabs.
32. **Chlorthalidone:** For hypertension 12.5–25 mg OD; as diuretic 50–100 mg OD in the morning. HYTHALTON 50, 100 mg tab., THALIZIDE 12.5, 25 mg tabs.
33. **Indapamide:** 2.5 mg OD; LORVAS, NATRILIX 2.5 mg tab, NATRILIX-SR, NATRITOR-SR 1.5 mg tab.
34. **Clonidine:** Start with 100 μg OD or BD, max 300 μg TDS, orally; CATAPRES 150 μg tab, ARKAMIN 100 μg tab.

35. Methyldopa: 0.25–0.5 g BD–QID; EMDOPA, ALPHADOPA 250 mg tab.
36. Hydralazine: 25–50 mg OD–TDS; NEPRESOL 25 mg tab.
37. Sodium nitroprusside: Initiate i.v. infusion with 0.02 mg/min, titrate with lowering of blood pressure upto 0.1–0.3 mg/min; SONIDE, PRUSIDE, NIPRESS 50 mg in 5 ml inj.

Note: *See* Index for preparations of other drugs.

Some combined antihypertensive formulations

1. Amlodipine 5 mg + Lisinopril 5 mg—AMLOPRES-L, LISTRIL-AM
2. Amlodipine 5 mg + Atenolol 50 mg—AMCARD-AT, AMLOPIN-AT, AMLOPRES-AT
3. Amlodipine 5 mg + Enalapril 5 mg—AMACE, AMTAS-E
4. Atenolol 25 mg or 50 mg + Chlorthalidone 12.5 mg—TENOCLOR, TENORIC
5. Enalapril 10 mg + Hydrochlorothiazide 25 mg–ENACE-D, VASONORM-H
6. Ramipril 2.5 mg + Hydrochlorothiazide 12.5 mg—CARDACE-H
7. Losartan 50 mg + Hydrochlorothiazide 12.5 mg—LOSAR-H, TOZAAR-H, LOSACAR-H
8. Lisinopril 5 mg + Hydrochlorothiazide 12.5 mg—LISTRIL PLUS, LISORIL-HT
9. Losartan 50 mg + Ramipril 2.5 mg or 5 mg—TOZAAR-R, LAPIDO-R
10. Losartan 50 mg + Amlodipine 5 mg—AMCARD-LP, AMLOPRES-Z, LOSACAR-A
11. Irbesartan 150 mg + Hydrochlorothiazide 12.5 mg—IROVEL-H, XARB-H.
12. Telmisartan 40 mg + Hydrochlorothiazide 12.5 mg—TELVAS-H, TELMA-H.

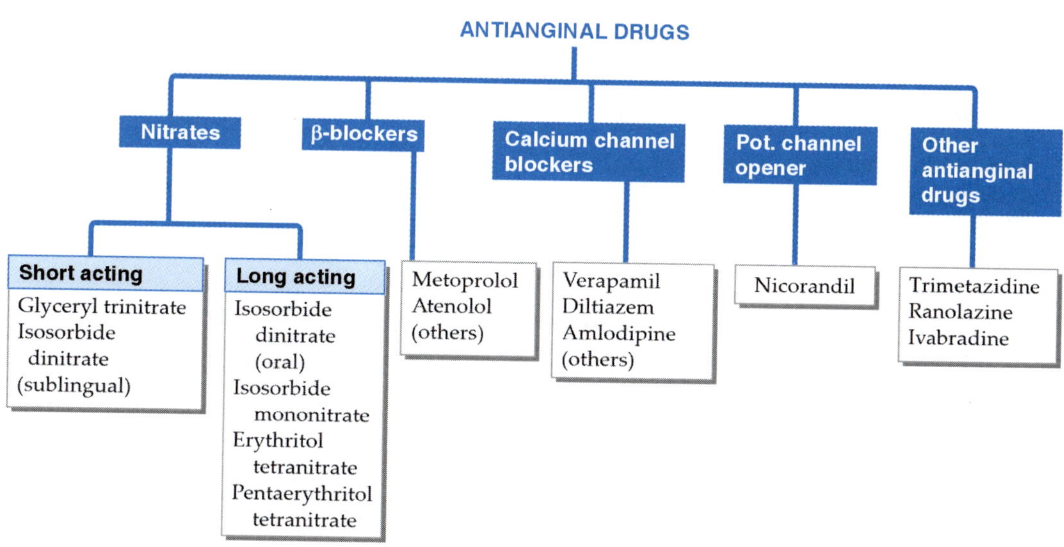
ANTIANGINAL DRUGS
Nitrates
β-blockers
Calcium channel blockers
Pot. channel opener
Other antianginal drugs
Short acting
Glyceryl trinitrate
Isosorbide dinitrate (sublingual)
Long acting
Isosorbide dinitrate (oral)
Isosorbide mononitrate
Erythritol tetranitrate
Pentaerythritol tetranitrate
Metoprolol
Atenolol
(others)
Verapamil
Diltiazem
Amlodipine
(others)
Nicorandil
Trimetazidine
Ranolazine
Ivabradine

Preparations

1. **Glyceryl trinitrate (GTN), Nitroglycerine:**
   0.5 mg sublingual, 0.4–0.8 mg s.l. spray; 5–15 mg oral;
   ANGISED 0.5 mg tab, NITROLINGUAL spray, GTN spray 0.4 mg per spray; ANGISPAN-TR 2.5, 6.5 mg SR cap, NITROCONTIN, CORODIL 2.6, 6.4 mg CR tabs.
   One transdermal patch for 14–16 hr per day; NITRODERM-TTS 5 or 10 mg patch;
   5–20 μg/min i.v.; MYOVIN, MILLISROL, NITROJECT 5 mg/ml inj.
2. **Isosorbide dinitrate:** 5–10 mg sublingual; SORBITRATE 5, 10 mg tab.
   10–20 mg oral; ISORDIL 5 mg sublingual & 10 mg oral tab; 20–40 mg sustained release oral.
3. **Isosorbide-5-mononitrate:** 10–40 mg oral; MONOTRATE 10, 20, 40 mg tab, 25 mg and 50 mg SR tab, 5-MONO, MONOSORBITRATE 10, 20, 40 mg tab.
4. **Erythrityl tetranitrate:** 15–60 mg oral; CARDILATE 5, 15 mg tab.
5. **Pentaerythritol tetranitrate:** 10–40 mg oral.
   PERITRATE 10 mg tab; 80 mg sustained release oral; PERITRATE-SA 80 mg SR tab.
6. **Nicorandil:** 5–20 mg BD.
   NIKORAN, 5, 10 mg tabs, 2 mg/vial and 48 mg/multidose vial inj; KORANDIL 5, 10 mg tabs.
7. **Trimetazidine:** 20 mg TDS after meals.
   FLAVEDON, CARVIDON, TRIVEDON 20 mg tabs, 35 mg modified release tab.
8. **Ranolazine:** 0.5–1.0 g BD as SR tab; RANOZEX, REVULANT, RANX, CARTINEX, RANOLAZ 500 mg SR tab.
9. **Ivabradine:** 5–7.5 mg BD, elderly 2.5 mg BD; IVABRAD, IVABEAT 5, 7.5 mg tab.

Note: See Index for preparations of β-blockers and calcium channel blockers.

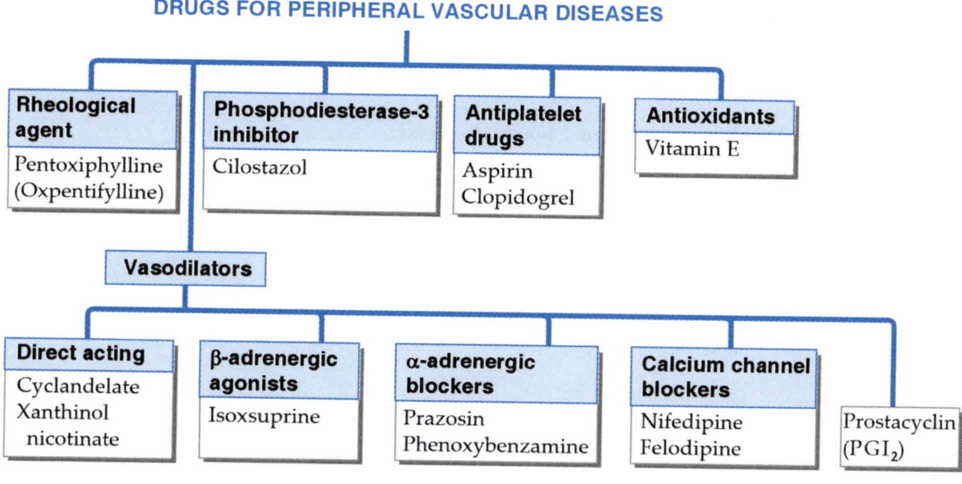
DRUGS FOR PERIPHERAL VASCULAR DISEASES
Rheological agent
Pentoxiphylline (Oxpentifylline)
Phosphodiesterase-3 inhibitor
Cilostazol
Antiplatelet drugs
Aspirin
Clopidogrel
Antioxidants
Vitamin E
Vasodilators
Direct acting
Cyclandelate
Xanthinol nicotinate
β-adrenergic agonists
Isoxsuprine
α-adrenergic blockers
Prazosin
Phenoxybenzamine
Calcium channel blockers
Nifedipine
Felodipine
Prostacyclin (PGI_2)

Preparations

1. **Pentoxiphylline:** 400 mg BD–TDS.
   TRENTAL-400, FLEXITAL 400 mg SR tab, 300 mg/15 ml for slow i.v. injection.
2. **Cyclandelate:** 200–400 mg TDS;
   CYCLOSPASMOL, CYCLASYN 200, 400 mg tab/cap.
3. **Xanthinol nicotinate:** 300–600 mg TDS oral; 300 mg by i.m. or slow i.v. injection;
   COMPLAMINA 150 mg tab, 500 mg retard tab, 300 mg/2 ml inj.
4. **Cilostazol:** 100 mg BD half hour before or 2 hours after food;
   CILODOC, PLETOZ, STILOZ, ZILAST 50, 100 mg tabs.

Note: *See* Index for preparations of other drugs.

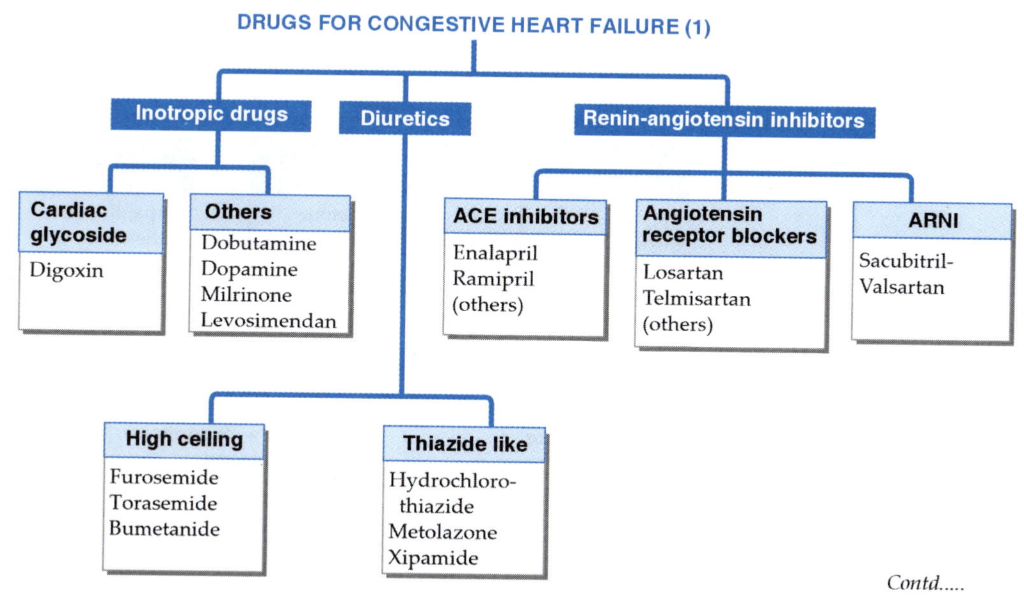

Contd.....

ACE: Angiotensin converting enzyme; ARNI: Angiotensin receptor-neprilysin inhibitor

Contd...

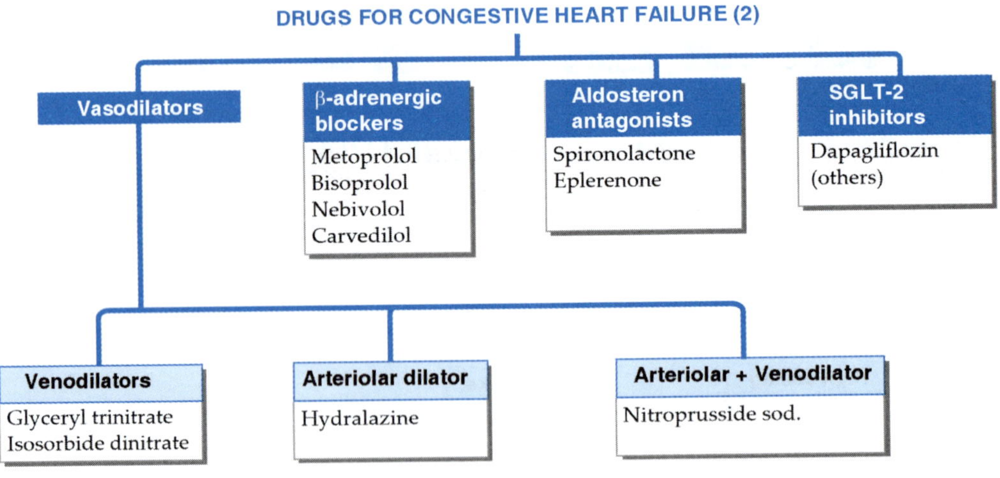

SGLT-2: Sodium-glucose cotransporter-2

Preparations

1. **Digoxin:** 0.25–0.5 mg/day (elderly 0.125–0.25 mg/day) oral adjusted according to response; 0.25 mg slow i.v. injection followed by 0.1 mg 1–2 hourly as needed; LANOXIN, SANGOXIN 0.25 mg tab, CELOXIN 0.25 mg tab, 0.05 mg/ml pediatric elixir, 0.5 mg/2 ml inj.
2. **Sacubitril-valsartan:** 50–200 mg/day oral; ENTRESTO, VYMADA 50, 100, 200 mg tabs (containing 24 + 26 mg, or 49 + 51 mg, or 97 + 103 mg sacubitril + valsartan).
3. **Milrinone:** 50 μg/kg i.v. bolus followed by 0.4–1.0 μg/kg/min i.v. infusion; PRIMACOR IV 10 mg/10 ml inj.

Note: *See* Index for preparations of other drugs.

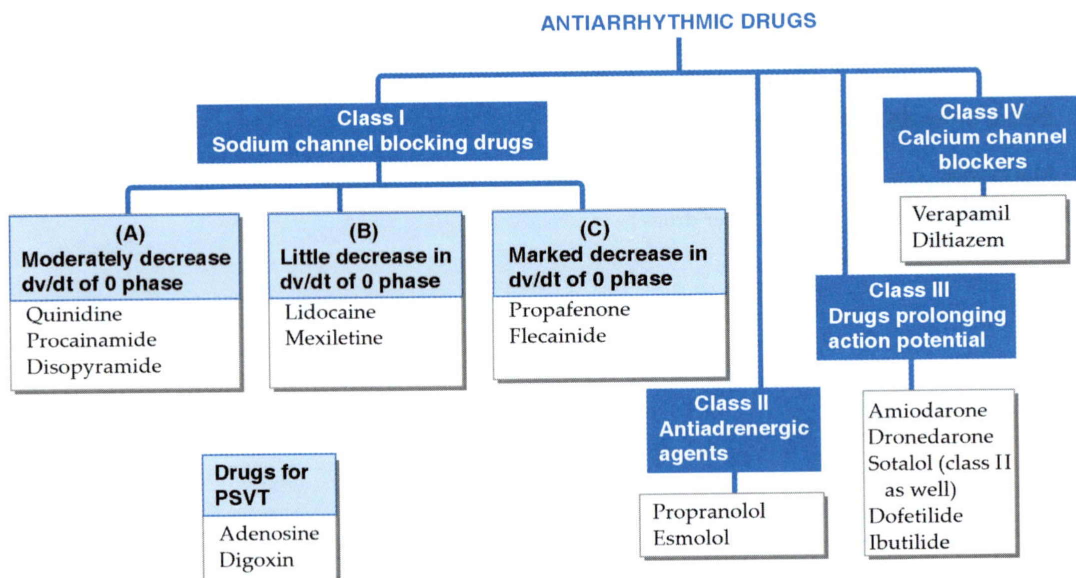

PSVT: Paroxysmal supraventricular tachycardia

Preparations

1. **Quinidine:** 100–200 mg TDS oral.
   QUINIDINE SULPHATE 200 mg tab; NATCARDINE 100 mg tab.
2. **Procainamide:** for abolition of arrhythmia—0.5–1 g oral or i.m. followed by 0.25–0.5 g every 2 hours; or 500 mg i.v. loading dose (25 mg/min injection) followed by 2mg/kg/hour.
   Maintenance dose—0.5 g every 4–6 hours;
   PRONESTYL 250 mg tab., 1 g/10 ml inj.
3. **Disopyramide:** 100–150 mg 6 hourly oral;
   NORPACE, 100, 150 mg cap, REGUBEAT 100 mg tab.
4. **Lidocaine (Lignocaine):** 50–100 mg i.v. bolus followed by 20–40 mg every 10–20 min or 1–3 mg/min i.v. infusion; XYLOCARD 20 mg/ml inj. (5, 50 ml vials). These preparations for cardiac use contain no preservative. The local anaesthetic preparations should not be used for this purpose.
5. **Mexiletine:** 100–250 mg i.v. over 10 min, 1 mg/min i.v. infusion; Oral: 150–200 mg TDS with meals;
   MEXITIL 50, 150 mg caps, 250 mg/10 ml inj.
6. **Propafenone:** 150 mg BD–300 mg TDS oral; RHYTHMONORM, PRADIL 150 mg tab.
7. **Propranolol:** 1 mg/min (max 5 mg) i.v. injection under close monitoring; 40–80 mg (max 160 mg) BD to QID oral; INDERAL, CIPLAR 10, 40, 80 mg tabs, 1 mg/ml inj, BETABLOCK 10, 40 mg tabs.
8. **Sotalol:** 40–80 mg BD–QID oral; SOTAGARD 40, 80 mg tabs, SOTALAR 40 mg tab.
9. **Esmolol:** 0.5 mg/kg in 1 min followed by 0.05–0.2 mg/kg/min i.v. infusion;
   MINIBLOCK 100 mg/10 ml, 250 mg/10 ml inj.
10. **Amiodarone:** 400–600 mg/day orally for few days, followed by 100–200 mg OD for maintenance; 100–300 mg (5 mg/kg) slow i.v. injection over 30–60 min;
    CORDARONE, ALDARONE, EURYTHMIC 100, 200 mg tabs, 150 mg/3 ml inj.

11. **Dronedarone:** 400 mg BD oral; MULTAQ, DILSAVE 400 mg tab.
12. **Verapamil:** 5 mg slow i.v. injection over 2–3 min (to terminate PSVT), 60–120 mg TDS orally for maintenance and to control ventricular rate in atrial fibrillation or flutter;
    CALAPTIN 40, 80 mg tab; 120, 240 mg SR tab, 5 mg/2 ml inj.
13. **Diltiazem:** 25 mg by slow i.v. inj (to terminate PSVT and to rapidly control ventricular rate in atrial fibrillation or flutter), 30–60 mg TDS orally for maintenance;
    DILZEM 30, 60 mg tabs, 90 mg SR tab; 25 mg/5 ml inj.
14. **Adenosine:** 6–12 mg (free base) by rapid i.v. injection in a central vein;
    ADENOJECT, ADENOCOR, 3 mg adenosine base per ml in 2 ml and 10 ml amp.
15. **Ivabradine:** For sinus tachycardia: 5 mg BD; increase to 7.5 mg BD if needed; elderly 2.5 mg BD;
    IVABEAT, IVABRAD, BRADIA 5, 7.5 mg tabs.

8 Drugs Acting on Kidney

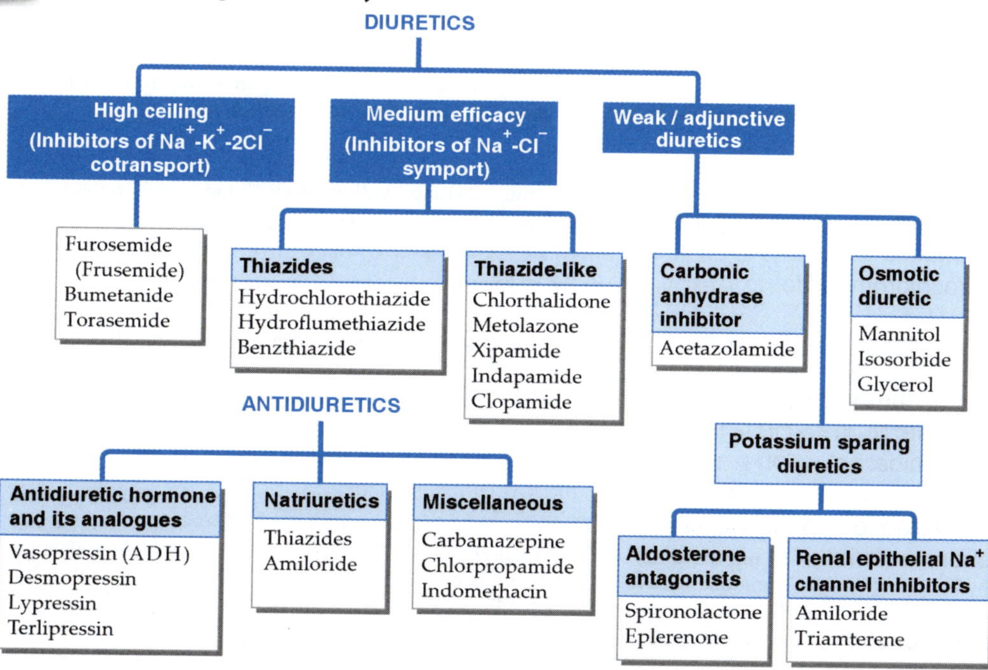

Preparations

Diuretics

1. **Furosemide (Frusemide):** Usual dose 20–80 mg orally once daily in the morning. In renal insufficiency, upto 200 mg 6 hourly may be given by i.m./i.v. route. In pulmonary edema 40–80 mg i.v.; LASIX 40 mg tab., 20 mg/2 ml inj. LASIX HIGH DOSE 500 mg tab, 250 mg/25 ml inj; (solution degrades spontaneously on exposure to light), SALINEX 40 mg tab, FRUSENEX 40, 100 mg tab.
2. **Bumetanide:** 1–5 mg oral once daily in the morning, 2–4 mg i.v./i.m. (max 15 mg/day in renal failure);
3. **Torasemide:** 2.5–20 mg once daily in the morning; upto 100 mg BD in renal failure; DIURETOR 10, 20 mg tabs, DYTOR, TIDE 5, 10, 20, 100 mg tabs, 10 mg/2 ml inj.
4. **Hydrochlorothiazide:** 12.5–100 mg OD in the morning; AQUAZIDE, THIAZIDE, HYDRIDE 12.5, 25, 50 mg tabs, ESIDREX 50 mg tab.
5. **Chlorthalidone:** As diuretic 50–100 mg OD in the morning; for hypertension 12.5–25 mg OD; HYTHALTON 50, 100 mg tab, THALIZIDE 12.5, 25 mg tabs.
6. **Metolazone:** 5–20 mg OD in the morning; DIUREM, METORAL 2.5, 5, 10 mg tabs.
7. **Xipamide:** 20–40 mg OD in the morning; XIPAMID 20 mg tab.
8. **Indapamide:** 2.5 mg OD in the morning; LORVAS, NATRILIX 2.5 mg tab; NATRILIX-SR 1.5 mg tab.
9. **Clopamide:** 10–60 mg OD in the morning; BRINALDIX 20 mg tab.
10. **Acetazolamide:** 250 mg OD–BD; DIAMOX, SYNOMAX 250 mg tab. IOPAR-SR 250 mg SR cap.
11. **Spironolactone:** 25–50 mg BD–QID; ALDACTONE 25, 50, 100 mg tabs; ALDACTIDE: Spironolactone 25 mg + hydroflumethiazide 25 mg tab; LACILACTONE, SPIROMIDE, Spironolactone 50 mg + furosemide 20 mg tab. TORLACTONE spironolactone 50 mg + torasemide 10 mg tab.
12. **Eplerenone:** 25–50 mg BD; EPTUS, EPLERAN, ALRISTA 25, 50 mg tabs.

13. **Triamterene:** 50–100 mg daily;
    DITIDE, triamterene 50 mg + benzthiazide 25 mg tab; FRUSEMENE, triamterene 50 mg + furosemide 20 mg tab.
14. **Amiloride:** 5–10 mg OD–BD;
    BIDURET, Amiloride 5 mg + hydrochlorothiazide 50 mg tab, LASIRIDE, AMIFRU amiloride 5 mg + furosemide 40 mg tab.
15. **Mannitol:** 100–500 ml of 10–20% solution infused i.v.;
    MANNITOL 10%, 20% in 100, 350 and 500 ml vac.

Antidiuretics

1. **Lypressin:** 10 IU i.m. or s.c., or 20 IU diluted in 100–200 ml of dextrose solution and infused i.v. over 10–20 min; PETRESIN, VASOPIN 20 IU/ml inj.
2. **Terlipressin:** 2 mg i.v., repeat 1–2 mg every 4–6 hours as needed;
   TERLINIS, T-PRESSIN 1 mg freez dried powder with 5 ml diluent for inj.
3. **Desmopressin (dDAVP):** *Intranasal:* Adults 10–40 μg/day in 2–3 divided doses, children 5–10 μg at bed time
   Oral: 0.1–0.2 mg TDS
   Parenteral (s.c. or i.v.) 2–4 μg/day in 2–3 divided doses.
   MINIRIN 100 μg/ml nasal spray (10 μg per actuation); 100 μg/ml intranasal solution in 2.5 ml bottle with applicator; 0.1 mg tablets; 4 μg/ml inj; D-VOID 100 μg/ml nasal spray.

9 Drugs Affecting Blood

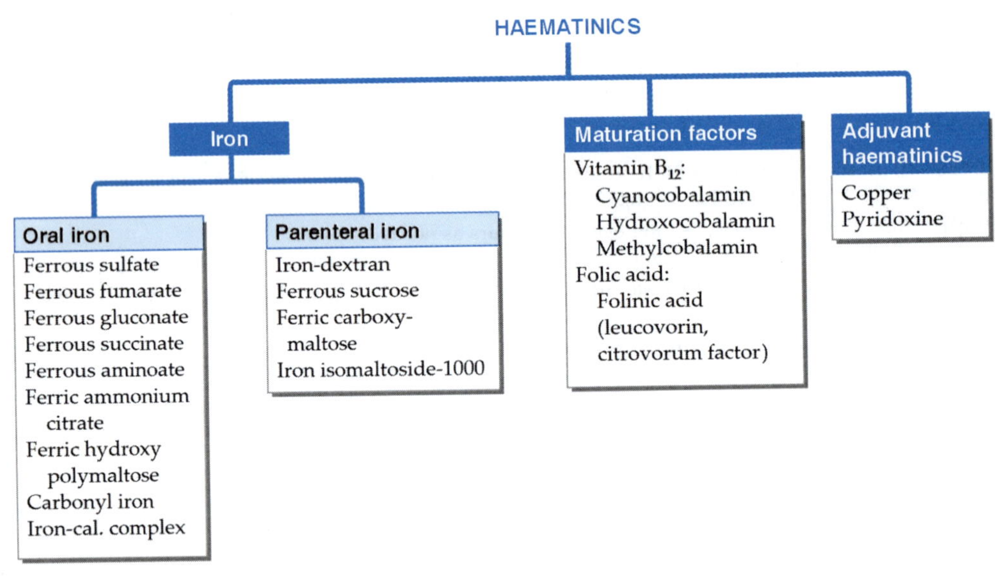

Preparations

Oral iron: Therapeutic dose: 100–200 mg elemental iron per day (children 3–5 mg/kg/day). Prophylactic dose: 30 mg elemental iron (children 1 mg/kg) per day.

1. Ferrous sulfate (hydrated salt 20% iron, dried salt 32% iron); FERSOLATE 200 mg tab.
2. Ferrous fumarate (33% iron); LOHTONE 300 mg cap.
3. Ferrous gluconate (12% iron).
4. Colloidal ferric hydroxide (50% iron); FERRI DROPS 50 mg/ml oral drops.

Combination oral iron preparations

Some combination preparations of iron

Trade name	Iron compound	Other ingredients
CONVIRON-TR Cap	Fe. sulfate (dried) 60 mg	B_{12} 15 μg, folic acid 1.5 mg, B_6 1.5 mg, vit. C 75 mg
FESOVIT-SPANSULE Cap	Fe. sulfate (dried) 150 mg	B_{12} 15 μg, folic acid 1 mg, nicotinamide 50 mg, B_6 2 mg
FERSOLATE-CM tab	Fe. sulfate (dried) 195 mg	Cu sulfate 2.6 mg, Mn. sulfate 2 mg
FEFOL Cap	Fe. sulfate 150 mg	Folic acid 0.5 mg
HEMGLOB syr (15 ml)	Fe. gluconate 300 mg	B_{12} 15 μg, B_1 5 mg, B_2 5 mg, B_6 1.5 mg, niacinamide 45 mg
AUTRIN Cap	Fe. fumarate 300 mg	B_{12} 15 μg, folic acid 1.5 mg
DUMASULES Cap	Fe. fumarate 300 mg	B_{12} 7.5 μg, folic acid 0.75 mg, B_1 5 mg, niacinamide 50 mg, vit. C 75 mg, B_6 1.5 mg
HEMSYNERAL-TD Cap	Fe. fumarate 200 mg	B_{12} 15 μg, folic acid 1.5 mg

Contd...

Contd...

HAEMUP GEMS Cap	Fe fumarate 200 mg	Folic acid 1.5 mg, Copper sulf. 2.5 mg, Mn. sulf 2.5 mg
HEMSI syr. (5 ml)	Fe. fumarate 100 mg	Vit B_{12} 5 μg, folic acid 0.5 mg, Zn 3.3 mg, Cu 0.035 mg, Mn 0.2 mg
FEFOL-Z Cap	Carbonyl iron (50 mg)	Folic acid 0.5 mg Zinc sulf. 22.5 mg
HBFAST tab	Carbonyl iron (100 mg iron)	Folic acid 0.35 mg
HEMATRINE Cap	Fe. succinate 100 mg	B_{12} 2.5 μg, folic acid 0.5 mg, vit. C 25 mg, niacinamide 15 mg
BIOFER tab POLYFER chewable tab	Ferric hydroxy polymaltose (Iron 100 mg)	Folic acid 0.35 mg
MUMFER syr (5 ml)	Ferric hydroxy polymaltose (50 mg iron)	
drops (1 ml)	—do—(50 mg iron)	
FERROCHELATE syr (5 ml)	Ferric ammon. cit. (Iron 60 mg)	B_{12} 5 μg, folic acid 1 mg
drops (1 ml)	—do—(Iron 20 mg)	B_{12} 4 μg, folic acid 0.2 mg
RARICAP tab	Iron cal. complex (Iron 25 mg)	Folic acid 0.3 mg
PROBOFEX Cap	Fe. aminoate (60 mg iron)	B_{12} 15 μg, folic acid 1.5 mg, B_6 3 mg
DEXORANGE Cap, syrup (15 ml)	Ferric ammon. cit. 160 mg	B_{12} 7.5 μg, folic acid 0.5 mg, Zn 7.5 mg (as sulfate)

Parenteral Iron

1. **Iron-dextran:** 50 mg elemental iron/ml in colloidal solution; 2 ml deep i.m. injection by 'Z' track technique, daily or on alternate days; 2 ml by slow i.v. injection (taking 10 min) daily;
   IMFERON, FERRI INJ: 100 mg in 2 ml amp.
2. **Ferrous-sucrose:** 100 mg slow i.v. inj. over 5 min daily or on alternate days. Not for i.m. or s.c. inj;
   MICROFER, UNIFERON, ICOR 50 mg in 2.5 ml and 100 mg in 5 ml inj.
3. **Ferric-carboxymaltose:** 100 mg slow i.v. inj. daily, or upto 1000 mg diluted in 100 ml saline and infused i.v. taking 15-30 min; infusion can be repeated after 1 week.
   ENCICARB INJ 50 mg/ml in 2 ml and 10 ml vials, OROFER FCM 500 mg/10 ml, 750 mg/15 ml, and 1000 mg/20 ml vial for inj.; dilute in 250 ml saline and infuse i.v. over 15–20 min.
4. **Iron isomaltoside-1000:** 100–200 mg i.v. over 5 min daily, or 1–2 g (max 20 mg/kg) i.v. infusion over 15–30 min;
   ISOFER, JILAZO 100 mg iron/ml inj in 1 ml and 5 ml vials.

Maturation factors

1. **Cyanocobalamin/Hydroxocobalamin:** Therapeutic dose: 30–1000 μg/day by i.m. or deep s.c. injection (not i.v.) for 10 days followed by weekly and then monthly doses; Prophylactic dose 3–10 μg/day oral; available only as combined formulations with other vitamins and iron:

   NEUROBION FORTE (1000 μg/3 ml inj; 15 μg per tab), OPTINEURON (1000 μg/3 ml inj), NEUROXIN-12 (500 μg/10 ml inj), POLYBION (15 μg per cap).
2. **Methylcobalamin:** 0.5–1.5 mg/day oral;
   BIOCOBAL, DIACOBAL, METHYCOBAL 0.5 mg tab, MECOBA, 0.5 mg tab and 0.5 mg in 1 ml inj.
3. **Folic acid:** Therapeutic dose 2–5 mg/day oral/i.m.; prophylactic dose 0.5 mg/day;
   FOLVITE, FOLITAB 5 mg tab.

4. **Folinic acid:** 1–3 mg i.v.; CALCIUM LEUCOVORIN 3 mg/ml inj; FASTOVORIN 3 mg and 15 mg amps, 50 mg vial; RECOVORIN 15 mg tab, 15 mg and 30 mg vial for inj.

Erythropoietic factor

1. **Recombinant human erythropoietin (Epoetin α, β):** 25–100 IU/kg s.c./i.v. 3 times a week (max 600 IU/kg/week);
   HEMAX 2000 IU/ml and 4000 IU/ml vials; EPREX 2000 IU, 4000 IU and 10,000 IU in 1 ml prefilled syringes; ZYROP (epoetin β) 2000 IU and 4000 IU vials.
2. **Darbepoetin α:** 0.45 μg/kg s.c. or i.v. once a week, adjust dose later according to rise in Hb level;
   CRESP 40 μg/vial inj.

COLONY STIMULATING FACTORS

Granulocyte colony stimulating factor (G-CSF)

1. **Filgrastim:** 5-10 μg/kg/day by slow i.v. infusion over 30 min, or by s.c. inj (for upto 2 weeks).
   CYTOGRAF, GRAFEEL, NEUPROGEN 300 μg/vial inj.
2. **Pegfilgrastim:** 6 mg s.c. once in each chemotherapy cycle.
   NEULASTIM, PEG-GRAFEEL 6 mg/vial inj.
3. **Lenograstim:** 150 μg/m^2/day s.c. inj. or infused i.v. over 30 min after dilution with saline, after 1 day of chemotherapy.
   GRAFEEL-PFS 300 μg prefilled syringe, GRANOCYTE 300 μg/vial inj.

Granulocyte-macrophage colony stimulating factor (GM-CSF)

1. **Sargramostim:** 250–500 μg/m^2/day by s.c. inj. or slow i.v. infusion.
   EMGRAST-M 500 μg/vial/inj.
2. **Molgramostim:** 5–10 μg/kg/day by s.c. inj. or slow i.v. infusion over 4 hours, starting 1 day after chemotherapy.
   LEUCOMAX 150 μg, 300 μg, 450 μg per vial inj.

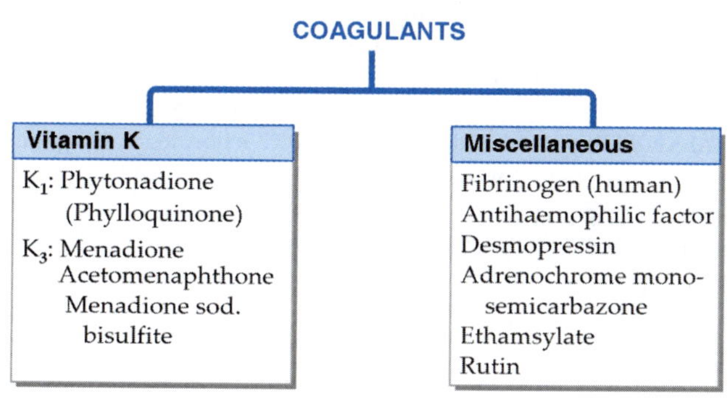

Preparations

1. **Vitamin K:** 5–10 mg oral/i.m., repeated as required;
   Phytonadione: VITAMIN-K, KENADION, K-WIN 10 mg/ml for i.m. injection.
   Menadione: 0.66 mg in GYNAE CVP with vit C 75 mg, ferrous gluconate 67 mg, cal. lactate 300 mg and citras bioflavonoid 150 mg per cap.
   Acetomenaphthone: ACETOMENADIONE 5, 10 mg tab; KAPILIN 10 mg tab.
   Menadione sod. bisulfite: STYPTOCID 10 mg with adrenochrome monosemicarbazone 0.5 mg, rutin 50 mg, vit C 37.5 mg, vit D 200 i.u., cal. phosphate 260 mg per tab.
2. **Fibrinogen:** 0.5 g by i.v. infusion; FIBRINAL 0.5 g Vac.
3. **Antihaemophilic factor:** 5–10 U/kg by i.v. infusion, repeated 6–12 hourly.
   FIBRINAL-H, ANTIHAEMOPHILIC FACTOR: 150 U or 200 U + fibrinogen 0.5 g/bottle for i.v. infusion.
4. **Rutin:** 60–200 mg BD–TDS oral; In CADISPER-C 60 mg tab.
5. **Ethamsylate:** 250–500 mg TDS oral/i.v.;
   ETHAMSYL, DICYNENE, HEMSYL 250, 500 mg tabs; 250 mg/2 ml inj.
6. **Desmopressin:** (*See* p. 113)

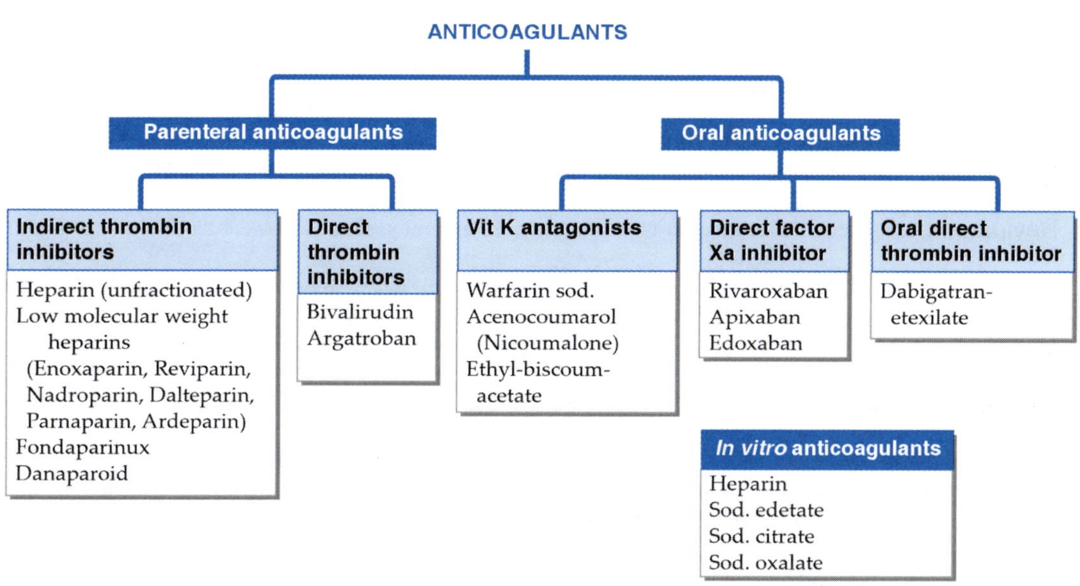
ANTICOAGULANTS
Parenteral anticoagulants
Oral anticoagulants
Indirect thrombin inhibitors
Heparin (unfractionated)
Low molecular weight heparins (Enoxaparin, Reviparin, Nadroparin, Dalteparin, Parnaparin, Ardeparin)
Fondaparinux
Danaparoid
Direct thrombin inhibitors
Bivalirudin
Argatroban
Vit K antagonists
Warfarin sod.
Acenocoumarol (Nicoumalone)
Ethyl-biscoum-acetate
Direct factor Xa inhibitor
Rivaroxaban
Apixaban
Edoxaban
Oral direct thrombin inhibitor
Dabigatran-etexilate
In vitro anticoagulants
Heparin
Sod. edetate
Sod. citrate
Sod. oxalate

Preparations

1. **Heparin (unfractionated):** 5000–10,000 U (children 50–100 U/kg) i.v. bolus dose followed by 750–1000 U/hr i.v. infusion;

   Low dose (s.c.) regimen: 5000 U s.c. every 8–12 hours;
   HEPARIN SOD., BEPARINE, NUPARIN 1000 and 5000 U/ml in 5 ml vials for injection.

2. **Low molecular weight (LMW) heparins:**

   Enoxaparin: CLEXANE 20 mg (0.2 ml) and 40 mg (0.4 ml) prefilled syringes; 20–40 mg OD, s.c. (start 2 hour before surgery).

   Reviparin: CLIVARINE 13.8 mg (eq. to 1432 anti Xa IU) in 0.25 ml prefilled syringe; 0.25 ml s.c. once daily for 5–10 days.

   Nadroparin: FRAXIPARINE 3075 IU (0.3 ml) and 4100 IU (0.4 ml) inj., CARDIOPARIN 4000 anti Xa IU/0.4 ml, 6000 anti Xa IU/0.6 ml, 100,000 anti Xa IU/10 ml inj.

   Dalteparin: 2500 IU s.c. OD for prophylaxis; 100 U/Kg 12 hourly or 200 U/Kg 24 hourly s.c. for treatment of deep vein thrombosis. FRAGMIN 2500, 5000 IU prefilled syringes.

   Parnaparin: 0.6 ml s.c. OD for unstable angina and prophylaxis of DVT; FLUXUM 3200 IU (0.3 ml), 6400 IU (0.6 ml) inj.

   Ardeparin: 2500–5000 IU s.c. OD; INDEPARIN 2500 IU, 5000 IU prefilled syringes.

3. **Fondaparinux:** 5–10 mg s.c. once daily for treatment of deep vein thrombosis (DVT)/pulmonary embolism (PE), 2.5–5 mg s.c. OD for prophylaxis of DVT/PE; FONDAPARINUX, ARIXTRA 5 mg/0.4 ml, 7.5 mg/0.6 ml and 10 mg/0.8 ml prefilled single dose syringe.

4. **Bivalirudin:** 0.75 mg/kg i.v injection, followed by 1.75 mg/kg/hour i.v. infusion for upto 24 hours; BIVAFLO, BIVASTAT, BIVASAVE 250 mg/vial inj.

5. **Argatroban:** 350 μg/kg i.v. inj. over 3–5 min, followed by 25 μg/kg/min i.v. infusion.
ARGATROBAN 100 mg/ml in 2.5 ml vials.
6. **Warfarin sod. (racemic):** 5–10 mg followed by 2–10 mg/day;
UNIWARFIN 1, 2, 5 mg tabs, WARF-5 5 mg tab.
7. **Acenocoumarol (Nicoumalone):** 8–12 mg followed by 2–8 mg/day; ACITROM 1, 2, 4 mg tabs.
8. **Rivaroxaban:** For prevention of DVT after knee/hip joint replacement 10 mg OD for 12–14 days (knee), 35 days (hip) replacement; 15 mg BD for treatment of DVT and PE; 2.5 mg OD with aspirin for prophylaxis of acute coronary syndrome.
XARELTO 2.5 mg, 10 mg, 15 mg, 20 mg tabs.
9. **Apixaban:** 2.5 mg BD for prophylaxis of DVT/PE following knee/hip replacement; 5 mg BD for prophylaxis of stroke in atrial fibrillation (AF) patients; 10 mg BD for 7 days followed by 5 mg BD for treatment of DVT/PE.
ELIQUIS 2.5 mg, 5 mg tabs.
10. **Edoxaban:** 60 mg OD; 30 mg OD for body weight <60 kg or Clcr <50 ml/min.
SAVAYSA 15, 30, 60 mg tabs.
11. **Dabigatran etexilate:** For prevention of venous thromboembolism following knee/hip replacement 110 mg OD (elderly >75 years 75 mg OD); 150 mg BD for prevention of stroke in AF patients;
PRADAXA 75, 110, 150 mg caps.
12. **Sodium citrate:** 1.65 g for 350 ml of blood (for transfusion); ANTICOAGULANT ACID CITRATE DEXTROSE SOLUTION 2.2 g/100 ml (75 ml is used for 1 unit of blood).
13. **Sodium oxalate:** 10 mg for 1 ml blood (for blood counts, etc.).
14. **Sodium edetate:** 2 mg for 1 ml blood (for investigations).

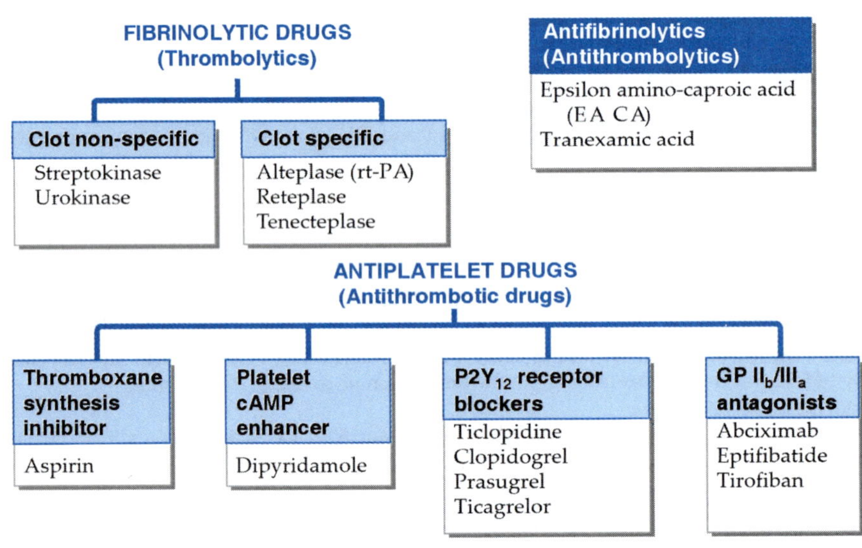
FIBRINOLYTIC DRUGS
(Thrombolytics)
Clot non-specific
Streptokinase
Urokinase
Clot specific
Alteplase (rt-PA)
Reteplase
Tenecteplase
Antifibrinolytics
(Antithrombolytics)
Epsilon amino-caproic acid
(EA CA)
Tranexamic acid
ANTIPLATELET DRUGS
(Antithrombotic drugs)
Thromboxane
synthesis
inhibitor
Aspirin
Platelet
cAMP
enhancer
Dipyridamole
P2Y12 receptor
blockers
Ticlopidine
Clopidogrel
Prasugrel
Ticagrelor
GP IIb/IIIa
antagonists
Abciximab
Eptifibatide
Tirofiban

Fibrinolytics

1. **Alteplase (recombinant tissue plasminogen activator (rt-PA):** *For MI:* 15 mg i.v. bolus injection followed by 50 mg over 30 min, then 35 mg over the next 1 hr. *For pulmonary embolism:* 100 mg i.v. infused over 2 hr. *For ischaemic stroke*: 0.9 mg/kg i.v. 10% of the dose injected in 1 min, remaining infused over 60 min; ACTILYSE 50 mg vial with 50 ml solvent water.
2. **Reteplase:** *For MI*: 18 mg (10 U) injected over 2 min, same dose repeated after 30 min; RETELEX 18 mg (10 U) per vial injection kit.
3. **Tenecteplase:** 0.5 mg/kg single i.v. bolus injection. ELAXIM 30 mg, 50 mg per vial inj.

Antifibrinolytics

1. **Epsilon amino-caproic acid (EACA):** Initial priming dose is 5 g oral/i.v., followed by 1 g hourly till bleeding stops (max. 30 g in 24 hrs).

   AMICAR, HEMOCID, HAMOSTAT 0.5 g tab., 1.25 g/5 ml syr., 5 g/20 ml inj.
2. **Tranexamic acid:** 10–15 mg/kg 2–3 times a day or 1–1.5 g TDS oral, 0.5–1 g TDS by slow i.v. infusion. DUBATRAN, PAUSE, TRANAREST 500 mg tab, 500 mg/5 ml inj., TRENAXA 500 mg tab.

Antiplatelet Drugs

1. **Aspirin:** 75–150 mg OD oral; COLSPRIN, DISPRIN CV–100: 100 mg soluble tab, LOPRIN 75 mg tab, ASPICOT 80 mg tab, ECOSPRIN 75, 150 mg tab.
2. **Dipyridamole:** 150–300 mg/day; PERSANTIN, 25 mg tab, THROMBONIL 75, 100 mg tabs; DYNASPRIN: dipyridamole 75 mg + aspirin 60 mg e.c. tab. CARDIWELL PLUS: dipyridamole 75 mg + aspirin 40 mg tab.

3. **Clopidogrel:** 300 mg loading dose followed by 75 mg daily; CLODREL, CLOPILET, DEPLATT 75 mg tab; Clopidogrel 75 mg + aspirin 75 mg: CLODREL PLUS, CLOPITAB-A, THROMBOSPRIN, SYNPLATT tab.
4. **Prasugrel:** Loading dose 60 mg followed by 10 mg OD: elderly and those below 60 kg body weight 5 mg OD; PRASULET, PRASUSAFE, PRASUREL 5 mg, 10 mg tabs.
5. **Ticagrelor:** 180 mg loading dose followed by 90 mg BD; BRILINTA, AXCER 90 mg tab. TICAPLAT 60 mg, 90 mg tab, TICAFLO 90 mg tab.
6. **Abciximab:** (Glycoprotein II_b/III_a receptor antagonist) 0.25 mg/kg i.v. 10–60 min before percutaneous coronary intervention (PTI), followed by 10 μg/min for 12 hr; REOPRO, FAXIMAB 2 mg/ml inj, 5 ml vial.
7. **Eptifibatide:** Initially 180 μg/kg/i.v. followed by 2 μg/kg/min i.v. infusion for upto 72 hours; CLOTIDE, EPTIFAB, UNIGRILIN, COROMAX 20 mg/10 ml and 75 mg/100 ml inj.
8. **Tirofiban:** Initially 0.4 μg/kg/min i.v. infusion for 30 min, followed by 0.1 μg/kg/min infusion for upto 48 hours. AGGRAMED, AGGRITOR, AGGRIBLOC 5 mg/100 ml infusion, TIROBAN 12.5 mg/50 ml and 5 mg/100 ml inj.

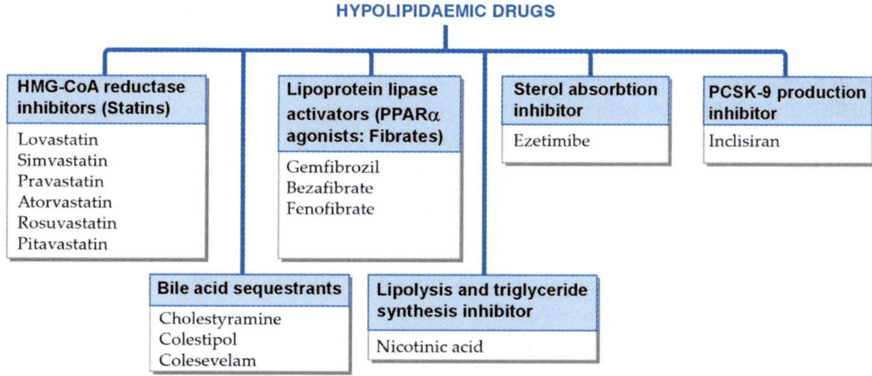

PCSK9: Proprotein convertase subtilisin-Kexin type 9

Preparations

1. **Lovastatin:** 10–40 mg/day; ROVACOR, AZTATIN, LOVAMEG 10, 20 mg tabs.
2. **Simvastatin:** 10–40 mg/day (max 80 mg, but high risk of myopathy); SIMVOTIN, SIMCARD, ZOSTA 5, 10, 20 mg tabs.
3. **Pravastatin:** 10–40 mg/day; PRAVATOR 10, 20 mg tabs.
4. **Atorvastatin:** 10–40 mg/day (max 80 mg); AZTOR, ATORVA, ATORLIP 5, 10, 20 mg tabs.

5. **Rosuvastatin:** 5–20 mg/day (max. 40 mg/day); ROSUVAS, ROSYN, ROZUTIN 5, 10, 20 mg tab.
6. **Pitavastatin:** 1–4 mg/day; PIVASTA 1, 2, 4 mg tabs. PITOSTAT 4 mg tab., PITASTAT 2 mg tab.
7. **Gemfibrozil:** 600 mg BD; GEMPAR, NORMOLIP, 300 mg cap., LOPID 300 mg cap, 600 mg tab.
8. **Bezafibrate:** 200 mg BD-TDS with meals; BEZALIP 200 mg tab, 400 mg SR (retard) tab.
9. **Fenofibrate:** 200 mg OD with meals; FENOLIP, LIPICARD 200 mg cap.
10. **Nicotinic acid:** Start with 100 mg TDS, gradually increase to 2–4 g per day in divided doses. It should be taken just after food to minimize flushing and itching;
    NIALIP, NEASYN-SR, 375, 500 mg tabs.
11. **Ezetimibe:** 10 mg OD; ZETICA, EZEDOC 10 mg tab.

    Ezetimibe 10 mg + atorvastatin 10 mg: BITORVA, LIPIVAS-EZ, LIPONORM-EZ;
    Ezetimibe 10 mg + simvastatin 10 mg: STARSTAT-EZ, SIMVAS-EZ.
12. **Inclisiran:** 284 mg s.c., next dose after 3 months, then one inj. every 6 months;
    SYBRAVA 284 mg/1.5 ml inj.

10 Gastrointestinal Drugs

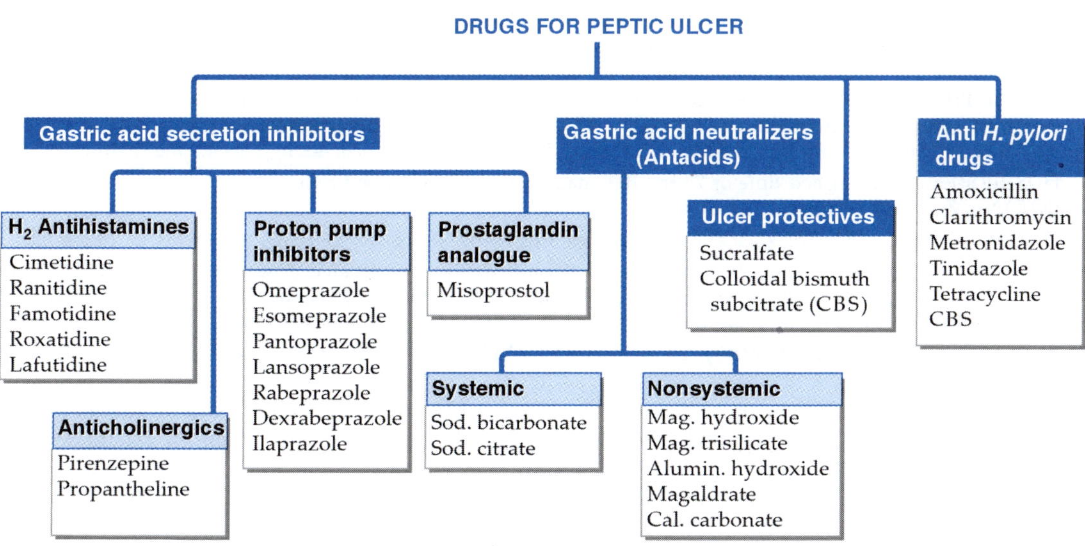

Preparations

1. **Ranitidine:** *For ulcer healing*—150 mg BD or 300 mg at bed time; *For prevention of ulcer recurrence*—150 mg at bed time; *For Zollinger-Ellison syndrome*—300 mg TDS or QID; *Parenteral dose for prevention of stress ulcer*—50 mg i.m. or slow i.v. injection every 6–8 hours or 0.1–0.25 mg/kg/hr i.v. infusion; ULTAC, ZINETAC 150 mg, 300 mg tabs; HISTAC, RANTAC, RANITIN, ACILOC 150 mg, 300 mg tabs, 50 mg/2 ml inj.
2. **Famotidine:** 40 mg at bed time or 20 mg BD (for healing); 20 mg at bed time for maintenance; upto 480 mg/day in ZE syndrome; parenteral dose 20 mg i.v. 12 hourly, or 2 mg/hr i.v. infusion.
   FAMTAC, FAMONITE, TOPCID 20 mg, 40 mg tabs; FAMOCID, FACID 20, 40 mg tabs, 20 mg/2 ml inj.
3. **Roxatidine:** 150 mg at bed time or 75 mg BD; maintenance 75 mg at bed time.
   ROTANE, ZORPEX 75 mg, 150 mg SR tabs.
4. **Lafutidine:** 10 mg after breakfast and after dinner; LAFAXID 10 mg tab, LAFTID, LAFUDAC 5, 10 mg tabs.
5. **Omeprazole:** 20–60 mg/day, ZE syndrome 60–120 mg/day in two divided doses; OMIZAC, NILSEC 20 mg cap. OMEZ, OCID, OMEZOL 10, 20 mg caps, PROTOLOC 20, 40 mg caps containing enteric coated granules. Capsules must not be opened or chewed; to be taken in the morning before meals, OCID, OMEZ 40 mg/amp inj.
6. **Esomeprazole (s-omeprazole):** 20–40 mg OD; NEXPRO, RACIPER, IZRA 20, 40 mg tab, RACIPER-IV 40 mg/5 ml inj.
7. **Lansoprazole:** Ulcer healing dose: 30 mg OD; LANZOL, LANZAP, LEVANT, LANPRO 15, 30 mg caps.
8. **Pantoprazole:** 40 mg OD; PANTOCID, PANTODAC 20, 40 mg enteric coated tab; PANTIUM, PANTIN 40 mg tab, 40 mg inj for i.v. use.
9. **S(-) Pantoprazole:** 20 mg OD; PANPURE, ZOSECTA 20 mg tab.
10. **Rabeprazole:** 20 mg OD, ZE syndrome 60 mg/day;
    RABLET, RAZO, RABELOC, RABICIP, HAPPI 10, 20 mg tab, 20 mg/ml for inj.
11. **Dexrabeprazole:** 10–20 mg OD; DEXPURE, 5, 10 mg tabs.

12. **Ilaprazole:** 5–20 mg OD before breakfast or before dinner; ILATOP, ILAGATE, ADIZA 5 mg, 10 mg tabs.
13. **Misoprostol (Methyl PGE_1 ester):** 200 μg QID; CYTOLOG 200 μg tab; MISOPROST 100 μg, 200 μg tabs.
14. **Magnesium hydroxide:** 0.4–1.0 g as often as required; MILK OF MAGNESIA 0.4 g/5 ml suspension.
15. **Aluminium hydroxide gel:** 0.6–2.4 g as required; ALUDROX 0.84 g tab, 0.6 g/10 ml suspension.
16. **Magaldrate:** 0.4–0.8 g as required; STACID 400 mg tab, 400 mg/5 ml susp;
    ULGEL 400 mg with 20 mg simethicone per tab or 5 ml susp.

    Combination antacid preparations

    ACIDIN: Mag. carb. 165 mg, dried alum. hydrox. gel 232 mg, cal. carb. 165 mg, sod. bicarb. 82 mg, with kaolin 105 mg and belladonna herb 30 μg per tab.

    ALMACARB: Dried alum. hydrox. gel 325 mg, mag. carb. 50 mg, methyl polysilox. 40 mg, deglycyrrhizinated liquorice 380 mg per tab.

    ALLUJEL-DF: Dried alum. hydrox. gel 400 mg, mag. hydrox. 400 mg, methyl polysilox. 30 mg per 10 ml susp.

    DIGENE GEL: Mag. hydrox. 185 mg, alum. hydrox. gel 830 mg, sod. carboxymethyl cellulose 100 mg, methylpolysilox. 25 mg per 10 ml susp.

    GELUSIL: Dried alum. hydrox. gel 250 mg, mag. trisilicate 500 mg per tab.

    GELUSIL LIQUID: Mag. trisilicate 625 mg, alum. hydrox. gel 312 mg per 5 ml susp.

    MUCAINE: Alum. hydrox. 290 mg, mag. hydrox. 98 mg, oxethazaine 10 mg per 5 ml susp.

    TRICAINE-MPS: Alum. hydrox. gel 300 mg, mag. hydrox. 150 mg, oxethazaine 10 mg, simethicone 10 mg per 5 ml gel.

    MAYLOX: Dried alum. hydrox. gel 225 mg, mag. hydrox. 200 mg, dimethicone 50 mg per tab and 5 ml susp.

    POLYCROL FORTE GEL: Mag. hydrox. 100 mg, dried alum. hydrox. gel 425 mg, methylpolysilox. 125 mg per 5 ml susp.
17. **Sucralfate:** Ulcer healing dose: 1 g taken 1 hour before 3 major meals and at bed time; To prevent recurrences 1 g BD; SUCRACE, ULCERFATE, RECULFATE 1 g tab.

18. **Colloidal bismuth subcitrate (CBS, Tripotassium dicitrato-bismuthate):** 120 mg (as Bi_2O_3) taken 30 min before 3 major meals and at bed time; TRYMO, DENOL 120 mg tab.

Anti-H. pylori antimicrobials

Amoxicillin: 750–1000 mg BD
Clarithromycin: 500 mg BD
Tetracycline: 500 mg QID
Metronidazole: 400 mg TDS
Tinidazole: 500 mg BD

Regimens consist of two of the above antimicrobials taken along with a proton pump inhibitor for 1–3 weeks.

Anti-*H. pylori* kits (one kit to be taken daily in 2 doses)

HP-KIT, HELIBACT, OMXITIN: Omeprazole 20 mg 2 cap + Amoxicillin 750 mg 2 tab + Tinidazole 500 mg 2 tab.
PYLOMOX: Lansoprazole 15 mg 2 cap + Amoxicillin 750 mg 2 tab + Tinidazole 500 mg 2 tab.
LANSI KIT: Lansoprazole 30 mg 1 cap + Amoxicillin 750 mg 1 tab + Tinidazole 500 mg 1 tab (one kit twice a day)
PYLOKIT, HELIGO: Lansoprazole 30 mg 2 cap + Clarithromycin 250 mg 2 cap + Tinidazole 500 mg 2 tab.
LANPRO AC: Lansoprazole 30 mg 2 cap + Clarithromycin 250 mg 2 tab + Amoxicillin 750 mg 2 tab.

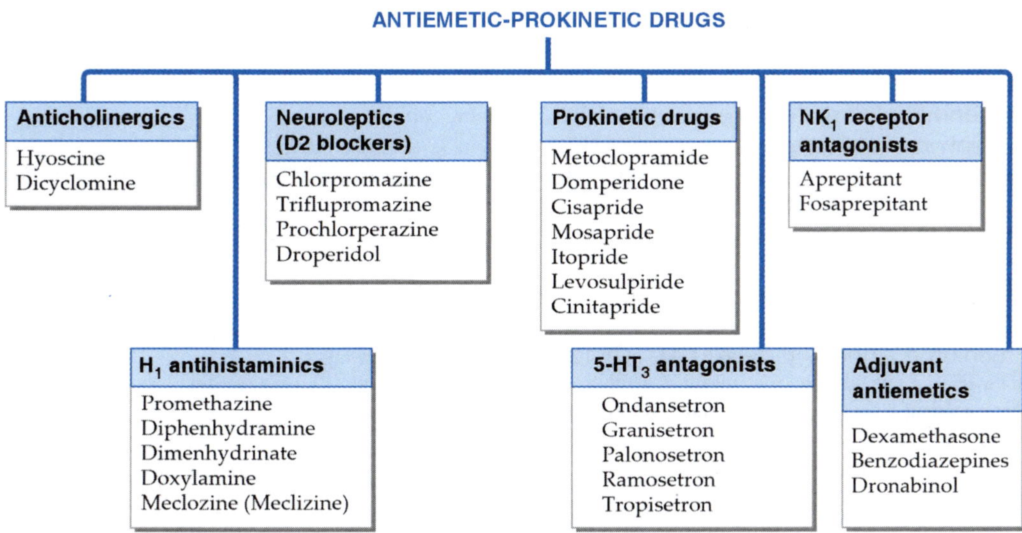
ANTIEMETIC-PROKINETIC DRUGS
Anticholinergics
Hyoscine
Dicyclomine
Neuroleptics (D2 blockers)
Chlorpromazine
Triflupromazine
Prochlorperazine
Droperidol
Prokinetic drugs
Metoclopramide
Domperidone
Cisapride
Mosapride
Itopride
Levosulpiride
Cinitapride
NK1 receptor antagonists
Aprepitant
Fosaprepitant
H1 antihistaminics
Promethazine
Diphenhydramine
Dimenhydrinate
Doxylamine
Meclozine (Meclizine)
5-HT3 antagonists
Ondansetron
Granisetron
Palonosetron
Ramosetron
Tropisetron
Adjuvant antiemetics
Dexamethasone
Benzodiazepines
Dronabinol

Preparations

1. **Hyoscine:** 0.2–0.4 mg oral/i.m./transdermal patch.
2. **Dicyclomine:** 10–20 mg oral/i.m.; CYCLOPAM 10 mg/ml inj in 2 ml and 10 ml amp/vial; COLIMEX, CYCLOPAM: dicyclomine 20 mg + paracetamol 500 mg tab.
3. **Promethazine theoclate:** 25–50 mg oral; AVOMINE 25 mg tab.
4. **Diphenhydramine:** 25–50 mg oral; BENADRYL 25, 50 mg cap.
5. **Dimenhydrinate:** 25–50 mg oral; DRAMAMINE 50 mg tab., 16 mg/5 ml sys.
6. **Meclozine:** 25–50 mg oral; PREGNIDOXIN: Meclozine 25 mg + caffeine 20 mg tab; DILIGAN: Meclozine 12.5 mg + nicotinic acid 50 mg tab.
7. **Doxylamine:** 10–20 mg at bed time (for morning sickness); DOXINATE, VOMNEX, NOSIC 10 mg tab (with pyridoxine 10 mg)
8. **Cinnarizine:** 25–50 mg oral; STUGE RON, VERTIGON 25 mg tab.
9. **Chlorpromazine:** 10–25 mg oral/i.m.
10. **Prochlorperazine:** 5–10 mg BD/TDS oral, 12.5–25 mg by deep i.m. inj.; STEMETIL 5 mg tab, 12.5 mg/ml inj in 1 ml amp, NAUSETIL 5 mg tab, 12.5 mg/ml inj.
11. **Droperidol:** 2.5 mg i.m. or i.v., followed by 1.25 mg when required. DROPEROL 2.5 mg in 1 ml inj.
12. **Metoclopramide:** 10 mg (children 0.25–0.5 mg/kg) TDS oral or i.m. For chemotherapy induced vomiting 0.3–2.0 mg/kg i.v./i.m;

    PERINORM, MAXERON, REGLAN, SIGMET, 10 mg tab; 5 mg/5 ml syr; 10 mg/2 ml inj.; 50 mg/10 ml inj.
13. **Domperidone:** 10–40 mg (Children 0.3–0.6 mg/kg) TDS; DOMSTAL, DOMPERON, NORMETIC 10 mg tab, 1 mg/ml susp, MOTINORM 10 mg tab, 10 mg/ml drops.

14. **Mosapride:** 5 mg (elderly 2.5 mg) TDS; MOZA, MOZASEF, MOPRIDE 2.5 mg, 5 mg tabs; MOZA MPS: 5 mg + methylpolysiloxane 125 mg tab.
15. **Itopride:** 50 mg TDS before meals; ITOKINE, ITOPRID, GANATON 50 mg tab.
16. **Levosulpiride:** 25 mg TDS to 75 mg twice daily as SR tab.;
    LESURIDE, NEXIPRIDE 25 mg tab, 75 mg SR tab, 25 mg/2 ml inj.
17. **Cinitapride:** 1 mg TDS 15 min before meals, or 3 mg OD as extended release (ER) tab;
    CINTAPRO, KINPRIDE, CIN MOVE 1 mg tab, 3 mg ER tab.
18. **Ondansetron:** For cisplatin and other highly emetogenic chemotherapy—8 mg i.v. by slow injection over 15 min, ½ hr before chemotherapeutic infusion, followed by 2 similar doses 4 hour apart. To prevent delayed emesis 8 mg oral is given twice a day for 3–5 days. For postoperative nausea/vomiting 4–8 mg i.v. given before induction is repeated 8 hourly. For less emetogenic drugs and for radiotherapy: oral dose of 8 mg is given 1–2 hr prior to the procedure and repeated twice 8 hrly.
    EMESET, VOMIZ, OSETRON, EMSETRON 4, 8 mg tabs, 2 mg/ml inj in 2 ml and 4 ml amps; ONDY, EMESET 2 mg/5 ml syr.
19. **Granisetron:** 1–3 mg diluted in 20–50 ml saline and infused i.v. over 5 min before chemotherapy, repeated after 12 hr. For less emetogenic regimen 2 mg oral 1 hr before chemotherapy or 1 mg before and 1 mg 12 hr after it. For post-operative vomiting 1 mg diluted in 5 ml and slowly injected i.v. followed by 1 mg orally every 12 hours.
    GRANICIP, GRANISET 1 mg, 2 mg tabs; 1 mg/ml inj. (1 ml and 3 ml amps).
20. **Palonosetron:** 250 μg by slow i.v. inj 30 min before chemotherapy; not to be repeated before 7 days. For post-operative vomiting 75 μg single injection. PALNOX 0.25 mg/ml inj; PALZEN 0.25 mg/50 ml inj.
21. **Ramosetron:** 0.3 mg i.v. before chemotherapy or surgery, may be repeated once daily, 0.1 mg oral for less emetogenic chemotherapy; NOZIA 0.1 mg tab, 0.3 mg in 2 ml amp.
22. **Tropisetron:** 5 mg i.v. just before chemotherapy, followed by 5 mg daily oral.
    TROPISETRON 1 mg/ml in 2 ml and 5 ml vials; 5 mg cap.

23. **Aprepitant:** 125 mg oral before chemotherapy and 80 mg on 2nd and 3rd day, alongwith i.v. ondansetron + dexamethasone. For postoperative vomiting 40 mg single oral dose before surgery;
APRECAP, APRISET, APRELIFE, EMPOV 125 mg (one cap) + 80 mg (2 caps) Kit.
24. **Fosaprepitant:** 150 mg i.v. over 20 min before chemotherapy (along with ondansetron + dexamethasone);
FOSARAN, EMOVID, FOSAPREPIT 150 mg/vial inj.
25. **Dexamethasone:** 8–20 mg i.v. 1/2–1 hour before emetogenic chemotherapy, generally to supplement metoclopramide/ondansetron.
26. **Diazepam:** 5–10 mg oral to supplement metoclopramide/ondansetron.
27. **Dronabinol:** 5–10 mg/m^2 body surface area orally for moderately emetogenic chemotherapy in patients non-responsive to other drugs.

Note: *See* Index for preparations of other drugs.

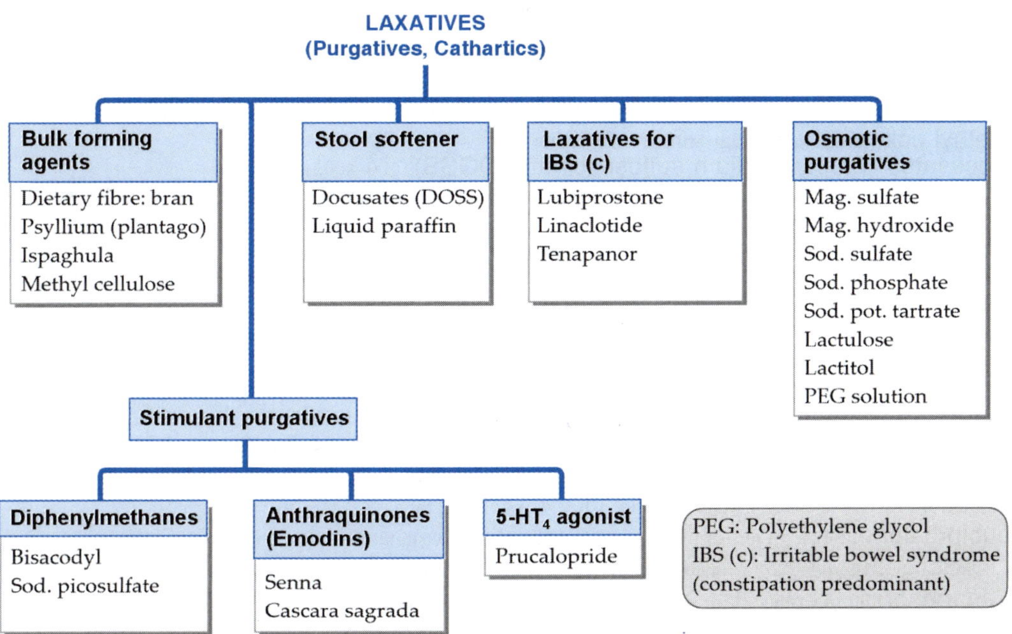
LAXATIVES
(Purgatives, Cathartics)
Bulk forming agents
Dietary fibre: bran
Psyllium (plantago)
Ispaghula
Methyl cellulose
Stool softener
Docusates (DOSS)
Liquid paraffin
Laxatives for IBS (c)
Lubiprostone
Linaclotide
Tenapanor
Osmotic purgatives
Mag. sulfate
Mag. hydroxide
Sod. sulfate
Sod. phosphate
Sod. pot. tartrate
Lactulose
Lactitol
PEG solution
Stimulant purgatives
Diphenylmethanes
Bisacodyl
Sod. picosulfate
Anthraquinones (Emodins)
Senna
Cascara sagrada
5-HT4 agonist
Prucalopride
PEG: Polyethylene glycol
IBS (c): Irritable bowel syndrome (constipation predominant)

Preparations

1. **Psyllium hydrophilic mucilloid:** 6–12 g to be taken just after mixing with water; ISOVAC 65 g/100 g granules.
2. **Ispaghula (refined husk):** 3–12 g freshly mixed with water or milk 2–3 times a day; ISOGEL (27 g/30 g), NATURE CARE (49 g/100 g), FYBOGEL (3.5 g/5.4 g) powder, FIBRIL (3.4 g/11 g) powder.
3. **Methyl cellulose:** 4–6 g/day mixed with water.
4. **Docusates (Dioctyl sodium sulfosuccinate, DOSS):** 100–400 mg/day; CELLUBRIL 100 mg cap; LAXICON 100 mg tab, DOSLAX 150 mg cap. As enema 50–150 mg in 50–100 ml; LAXICON 125 mg in 50 ml enema.
5. **Liquid paraffin:** 15–30 ml/day as such or in emulsified form; AGAROL: 4.8 ml with glycine and sorbitol in 15 ml aqueous emulsion, CREMAFFIN: Liq. paraffin 3.75 ml with milk of magnesia 11.25 ml/15 ml emulsion.
6. **Bisacodyl:** 5–10 mg oral at bed time; DULCOLAX 5 mg tab; 10 mg (adult) 5 mg (child) suppository in the morning. CONLAX 5 mg, 10 mg suppository.
7. **Sodium picosulfate:** 5-10 mg at bed time; CREMALAX, LAXICARE 10 mg tab, PICOFATE 5 mg/5 ml syr.
8. **Senna (as Sennosides Cal. salt):** 10–40 mg at bed time: GLAXENNA 11.5 mg tab; SOFSENA 12 mg tab, EVACUOL GRANULES 18 mg/dose.
9. **Prucalopride:** 2 mg once daily; elderly—start with 1 mg OD; PRUEASE, PRESMOVAC, PRUMAX, PRUVICT 1 mg, 2 mg tabs.
10. **Lubiprostone:** 24 μg BD with meals; LUBOWEL 24 μg soft gelatin caps.
11. **Linaclotide:** 145 μg–290 μg once daily oral. LINZESS 145 μg and 290 μg caps.
12. **Tenapanor:** 50 mg twice daily before breakfast and dinner. IBSRELA 50 mg tab.

13. **Mag. sulfate (Epsom salt):** 5–15 g dissolved in 150–200 ml water, taken in the morning.
14. **Mag. hydroxide** (as 8% W/W suspension—milk of magnesia) 30 ml taken early morning.
15. **Sod. sulfate (Glauber's salt):** 10–15 g dissolved in 150–200 ml water, taken in the morning.
16. **Sod. phosphate:** 6–12 g dissolved in 150–200 ml water, taken in the morning.
17. **Sod. pot. tartrate (Rochelle salt):** 8–15 g dissolved in 150–200 ml water, taken in the morning.
18. **Lactulose:** 10 g BD taken with water;
    LACSAN 10 g/15 ml liquid, DUPHALAC, LIVOLUK 6.67 g/10 ml liq; LOOZ 10 g/15 ml soln.
19. **Lactitol:** 10–20 g as syrup containing 10 g/15 ml; or as granules dissolved in water;
    LACTIHEP, GUTCLEAR, EVA-Q: lactitol 10 g/15 ml syr, 10 g granules sachet,
    CADILOSE GREEN GRANULES: lactitol 10 g + ispaghula husk 3.5 g/15 g sachet.

Some combined preparations

CREMAFFIN: Milk of magnesia 11.25 ml, liq. paraffin 3.75 ml per 15 ml emulsion.
JULAX: Bisacodyl 10 mg, casanthranol 10 mg dragees.
PURSENNID-IN (with DOS): Purified senna ext. (cal salt) 18 mg, docusates 50 mg tab.

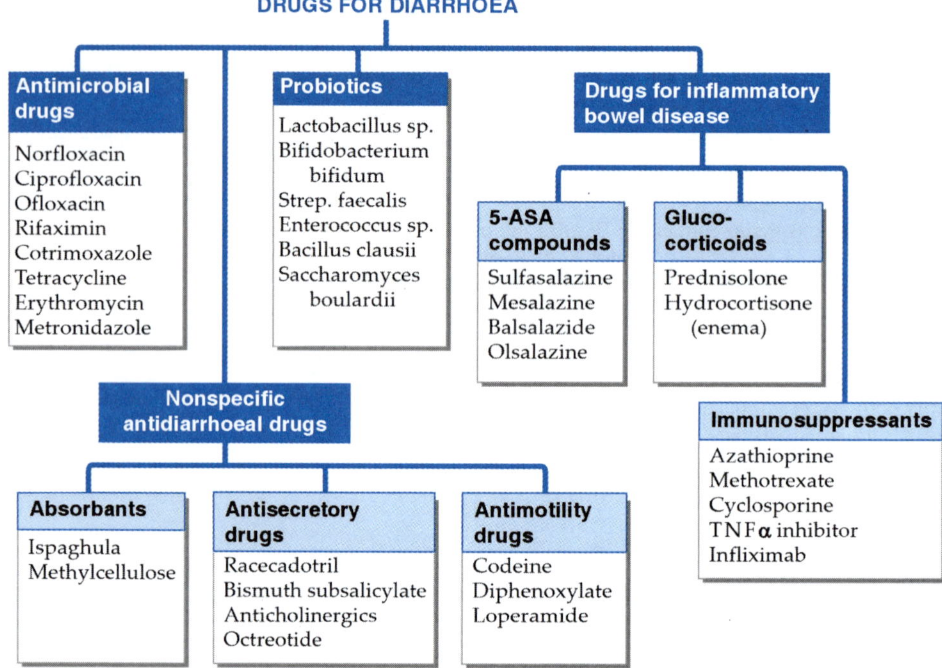
DRUGS FOR DIARRHOEA
Antimicrobial drugs
Norfloxacin
Ciprofloxacin
Ofloxacin
Rifaximin
Cotrimoxazole
Tetracycline
Erythromycin
Metronidazole
Probiotics
Lactobacillus sp.
Bifidobacterium bifidum
Strep. faecalis
Enterococcus sp.
Bacillus clausii
Saccharomyces boulardii
Drugs for inflammatory bowel disease
5-ASA compounds
Sulfasalazine
Mesalazine
Balsalazide
Olsalazine
Gluco-corticoids
Prednisolone
Hydrocortisone (enema)
Immunosuppressants
Azathioprine
Methotrexate
Cyclosporine
TNFα inhibitor
Infliximab
Nonspecific antidiarrhoeal drugs
Absorbants
Ispaghula
Methylcellulose
Antisecretory drugs
Racecadotril
Bismuth subsalicylate
Anticholinergics
Octreotide
Antimotility drugs
Codeine
Diphenoxylate
Loperamide

Preparations

1. **Rifaximin:** For traveller's diarrhoea 200–400 mg TDS for 3 days. For suppressing ammonia forming gut bacteria 550 mg TDS; RIFAGUT, TORFIX 200 mg, 400 mg tabs. RIXIMIN 200, 400, 550 mg tabs.
2. **Probiotics:**
   - ECONORM, STIBS: *Saccharomyces boulardii* 250 mg sachet.
   - DAROLAC: *Lactobacillus, B. longam, S. boulardii* 1.25 billion (B) live cells/sachet; One sachet to be suspended in milk, water or fruit juice and taken once a day.
   - BIFILAC: *Lactobacillus* 50 million (M), *Streptococcus faecalis* 30M, *Clostridium butyricum* 2M, *Bacillus mesentericus* 1M per cap/sachet.
   - BIFILIN: *Lactobacillus sp.* 1 billion (B), *Bifidobacterium bifidum* 1B, *Streptococcus thermophillus* 0.25B, *Saccharomyces boulardii* 0.25B per cap and sachet.
   - ACTIGUT: *Lactobacillus sp., Bifidobacterium sp.* cap.
   - ENTEROGERMINA: *Bacillus claussi* 2B spores/5 ml oral amp.
3. **Racecadotril:** 100 mg (children 1.5 mg/kg) TDS for a maximum of 7 days; CADOTRIL, RACIGYL 100 mg cap, 15 mg sachet, REDOTIL 100 mg cap, ZEDOTT, ZOMATRIL 100 mg tab., 10 mg and 30 mg sachets and dispersible tabs.
4. **Codeine:** 60 mg TDS oral.
5. **Diphenoxylate-atropine:** LOMOTIL 2.5 mg diphenoxylate + 0.025 mg atropine per tab and 5 ml liquid; 2–4 tab followed by 1–2 tab 6 hourly.
6. **Loperamide:** 4 mg followed by 2 mg after each motion (max. 10 mg in a day); 2 mg BD for chronic diarrhoea. IMODIUM, LOPAMIDE, DIARLOP: 2 mg tab, cap.
7. **Sulfasalazine (Salicylazosulfapyridine):** For inflammatory bowel disease—Remission inducing dose 3–4 g/day, maintenance dose 1.5–2 g/day oral; SALAZOPYRIN, SALAZAR, SAZO-EN 0.5 g tab.
8. **Mesalazine (Mesalamine):** 1.2–2.4 g/day oral; 4 g by retention enema; MESACOL 0.4 g and 0.8 g tab, 0.5 g suppository; ASACOL, TIDOCOL 0.4 g tab, MESACOL ENEMA 4 g/60 ml.
9. **Balsalazide:** 1.5 g BD-2.25 g TDS; COLOREX 750 mg cap and per 5 ml syr., INTAZIDE, BALACOL 0.75 g tab.

Note: *See* Index for preparations of other drugs

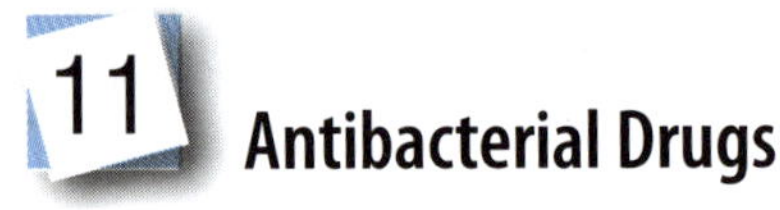

11 Antibacterial Drugs

ANTIBACTERIAL DRUGS

Inhibit cell wall synthesis
- Penicillins
- Cephalosporins
- Carbapenems
- Monobactams
- Vancomycin
- Cycloserine
- Bacitracin

Cause leakage from cell membranes
- Polymyxin
- Colistin
- Bacitracin
- Amphotericin B

Inhibit protein synthesis
- Tetracyclines
- Chloramphenicol
- Erythromycin (other macrolides)
- Clindamycin
- Linezolid

Cause misreading of m-RNA → affect permeability
- Aminoglycosides: (Streptomycin, Gentamicin, others)

Inhibit DNA gyrase
- Ciprofloxacin (Other fluoroquinolones)

Interfere with DNA function
- Rifampin

Interfere with intermediary metabolism
- Sulfonamides
- Sulfones
- Trimethoprim
- Pyrimethamine
- Para amino-salicylic acid
- Metronidazole

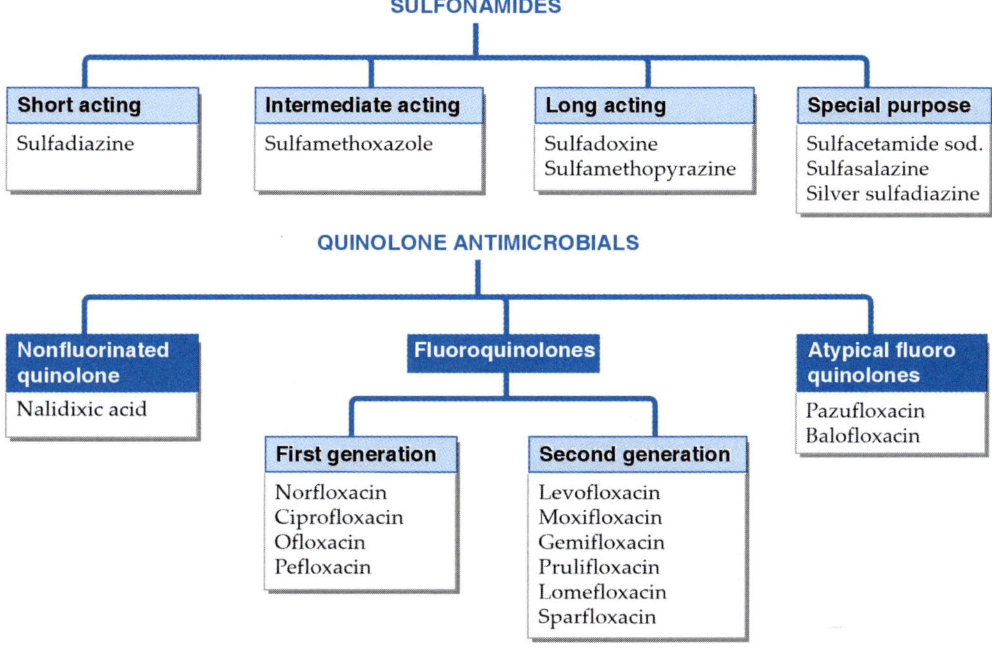
SULFONAMIDES
Short acting
Sulfadiazine
Intermediate acting
Sulfamethoxazole
Long acting
Sulfadoxine
Sulfamethopyrazine
Special purpose
Sulfacetamide sod.
Sulfasalazine
Silver sulfadiazine
QUINOLONE ANTIMICROBIALS
Nonfluorinated quinolone
Nalidixic acid
Fluoroquinolones
First generation
Norfloxacin
Ciprofloxacin
Ofloxacin
Pefloxacin
Second generation
Levofloxacin
Moxifloxacin
Gemifloxacin
Prulifloxacin
Lomefloxacin
Sparfloxacin
Atypical fluoro quinolones
Pazufloxacin
Balofloxacin

Preparations

Sulfonamides

1. **Sulfadiazine:** 0.5–2.0 g TDS.
2. **Sulfamethoxazole:** 1 g BD for 2 days, then 0.5 g BD.
3. **Sulfacetamide sodium:** 6%–30% topically in the eye;
   LOCULA, ALBUCID 10%, 20%, 30% eye drops, 6% eye oint.
4. **Silver sulfadiazine:** 1% topical application;
   SILVIRIN 1% cream, ARGISEPT 1% cream with chlorhexidine 0.2%.

Note: See Index for preparations of other sulfonamides.

Cotrimoxazole

(Trimethoprim-Sulfamethoxazole 1:5)

SEPMAX, CIPLIN, ORIPRIM, SUPRISTOL, FORTRIM

Trimethoprim	*Sulfamethoxazole*
80 mg +	400 mg tab: 2 BD for 2 days then 1 BD.
160 mg +	800 mg tab: double strength (DS); 1 BD.
20 mg +	100 mg pediatric tab.
40 mg +	200 mg per 5 ml susp; infant 2.5 ml (not to be used in new borns), children 1–5 yr 5 ml, 6–12 year 10 ml (all BD).

Quinolones Antimicrobials

1. **Nalidixic acid:** 0.5–1 g TDS or QID oral; GRAMONEG 0.5 g tab, 0.3 g/5 ml susp.
2. **Ciprofloxacin:** 250–750 mg BD oral, 100–200 mg i.v. by slow infusion; 0.3% topically in eye; CIFRAN, CIPLOX, CIPROBID, QUINTOR, CIPROLET 250, 500, 750 mg tab, 200 mg/100 ml i.v. infusion, 3 mg/ml eye drops.
3. **Ofloxacin:** 200–400 mg BD oral, 200 mg by slow i.v. infusion; 0.3% topically in eye; ZANOCIN, TARIVID, OFLOX 100, 200, 400 mg tab; 200 mg/100 ml i.v. infusion, ZENFLOX also 50 mg/5 ml susp., EXOCIN, OFLOX 0.3% eye drops.
4. **Norfloxacin:** 200–400 mg BD oral, 0.3% topically in eye; NORBACTIN, NORFLOX 200, 400, 800 mg tab, 3 mg/ml eye drops. UROFLOX, NORILET 200, 400 mg tab, BACIGYL Norfloxacin 100 + metronidazole 100 mg/5 ml syrup.
5. **Pefloxacin:** 400 mg BD oral, 400 mg i.v. by slow infusion; PELOX 200, 400 mg tab, to be taken with meals; 400 mg/5 ml inj (to be diluted in 100–250 ml of glucose solution but not saline).
6. **Levofloxacin:** 500 mg OD oral, 500 mg by slow i.v. infusion; TAVANIC, LEVOFLOX, LEVODAY, GLEVO 250, 500 mg tab, 500 mg/100 ml inj, GLEVO 0.5% eye drops.
7. **Lomefloxacin:** 400 mg OD oral; LOMEF–400, LOMEDON, LOMADAY 400 mg tab., LOMIBACT, LOX 400 mg tab, 0.3% eye drops.
8. **Sparfloxacin:** 200–400 mg OD oral; TOROSPAR 200, 400 mg tab, SPARTA, SPARQUIN, SPARDAC 100, 200 mg tab, ZOSPAR, EYPAR 0.3% eye drops.
9. **Moxifloxacin:** 400 mg OD oral; MOXIF, MOXICIP 400 mg tab, STAXOM 400 mg tab, 400 mg/250 ml i.v. infusion, VIGAMOX, MOXICIP 0.5% eye drops.
10. **Gemifloxacin:** 320 mg OD for 5-7 days; TOPGEM, GEMI, GEMBAX, GEMISTAR 320 mg tab.
11. **Prulifloxacin:** 600 mg OD; ALPRULI, PRULIFACT 600 mg tab.
12. **Pazufloxacin:** 500 mg (elderly 300 mg) infused i.v. over 30–60 min twice daily; PAZACE, PAZFLO, PAZUBID 500 mg/100 ml and 300 mg/100 ml inj.
13. **Balofloxacin:** 100–200 mg BD; BALOXIN, BALOWIN, B-CIN 100 mg tab.

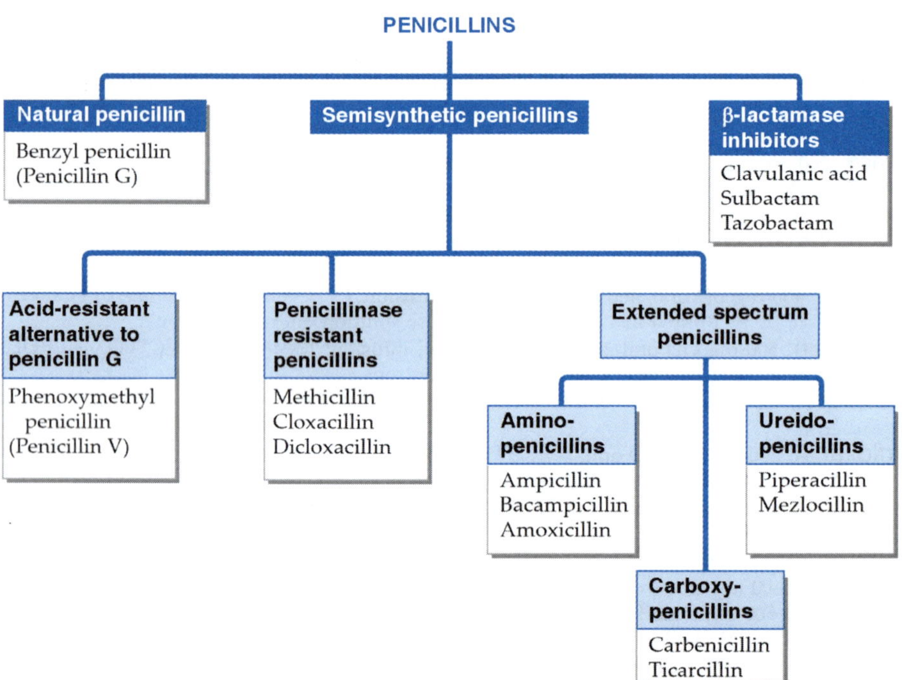
PENICILLINS
Natural penicillin
Benzyl penicillin
(Penicillin G)
Semisynthetic penicillins
β-lactamase inhibitors
Clavulanic acid
Sulbactam
Tazobactam
Acid-resistant alternative to penicillin G
Phenoxymethyl penicillin
(Penicillin V)
Penicillinase resistant penicillins
Methicillin
Cloxacillin
Dicloxacillin
Extended spectrum penicillins
Amino-penicillins
Ampicillin
Bacampicillin
Amoxicillin
Ureido-penicillins
Piperacillin
Mezlocillin
Carboxy-penicillins
Carbenicillin
Ticarcillin

Preparations

1. **Sod. penicillin G (crystalline penicillin) injection:** 0.5–5 MU i.m./i.v. 6–12 hourly. BENZYL PENICILLIN 0.5, 1.0 MU dry powder in vial to be dissolved in sterile water at the time of injection.
2. **Fortified procaine penicillin G inj:** contains 3 lac U procaine penicillin and 1 lac U sod. penicillin G, FORTIFIED P.P. INJ 3+1 lac U vial; BISTREPEN 6 + 4 lakh U/vial inj.
3. **Benzathine penicillin G:** 0.6–2.4 MU i.m. every 2–4 weeks as aqueous suspension. PENIDURE-LA (long acting), LONGACILLIN, 0.6, 1.2, 2.4 MU as dry powder in vial.
4. **Phenoxymethyl penicillin (Penicillin V):** Adults 250–500 mg, infants 60 mg, children 125–250 mg; given 6 hourly, (250 mg = 4 lac U); KAY PEN 125 mg, 250 mg tabs.
5. **Cloxacillin / dicloxacillin:** 0.25–0.5 g orally every 6 hours; for severe infections 0.5–1 g may be injected i.m. or i.v.; KLOX, BIOCLOX, 0.25, 0.5 g cap; 0.25, 0.5 g/vial inj. JOLCLO 0.5 g, 1.0 g/vial powder for injection.
6. **Ampicillin:** 0.5–2 g oral/i.m./i.v. depending on severity of infection, every 6–8 hours; children 50–100 mg/kg/day; AMPILIN, ROSCILLIN, BIOCILIN 250, 500 mg cap; 125, 250 mg/5 ml dry syr; 100 mg/ml pediatric drops; 250, 500 mg and 1.0 g per vial inj. AMPILONG-DS: ampicillin 0.5 g + probenecid 0.5 g tab.
7. **Bacampicillin:** 400–800 mg BD oral; PENGLOBE 200, 400 mg tabs.
8. **Amoxicillin:** 0.25–1 g TDS oral/i.m or slow i.v. injection, children 25–75 mg/kg/day; AMOXYPEN, NOVAMOX, SYNAMOX 250, 500 mg cap, 125 mg/5 ml dry syr; AMOXIL, MOX 250, 500 mg caps; 125 mg/5 ml dry syr; 250, 500 mg/vial inj. MOXYLONG: Amoxicillin 250 mg + probenecid 500 mg tab (also 500 mg + 500 mg DS tab).
9. **Amoxicillin + Cloxacillin:** NOVACLOX 250 + 250 mg cap, 125 + 125 mg pediatric tab, 125 + 125 mg inj, 250 + 250 mg inj, 500 + 500 mg inj.; 50 + 25 mg neonatal inj.
10. **Carbenicillin:** 1–2 g i.m. or 1–5 g i.v. 4–6 hourly; CARBELIN 1.0 g, 5.0 g per vial inj.

11. **Ticarcillin:** 3 g i.m./i.v. 6 hourly;
TIMENTIN: Ticarcillin disod. + clavulanate pot. 3.1 g/vial powder for reconstitution before injection.

12. **Piperacillin:** 100–150 mg/kg/day in 3 divided doses (max 16 g/day) i.m. or i.v. The i.v. route is preferred when > 2 g is to be injected.
PIPRAPEN 1 g, 2 g vials; PIPRACIL 2 g, 4 g vials for inj; contains 2 mEq Na^+ per g.

13. **Amoxicillin + Clavulanic acid (co-amoxiclav):** AUGMENTIN, ENHANCIN, AMONATE: Amoxicillin 250 mg + clavulanic acid 125 mg tab, also 500 + 125 mg tab, 125 mg + 31.5 mg per 5 ml dry syr; 1–2 tab TDS, severe infections 4 tabs 6 hourly; CLAVAM 250 + 125 mg tab, 500 + 125 mg tab, 875 + 125 mg tab, 125 mg + 32 mg per 5 ml dry syr.
Also AUGMENTIN, CLAVAM INJ; Amoxicillin 1 g + clavulanic acid 0.2 g vial and 0.5 g + 0.1 g vial; inject 1 vial deep i.m. or i.v. 6–8 hourly for severe infections.

14. **Ampicillin + Sulbactam:** SULBACT, AMPITUM: Ampicillin 1 g + sulbactam 0.5 g per vial inj; 1–2 vial deep i.m. or i.v. injection 6–8 hourly.

15. **Sultamicillin tosylate (a complex salt of ampicillin and sulbactam):**
SULBACIN 375 mg tab, BACTOMIN 375 mg, 750 mg tab.

16. **Piperacillin + Tazobactam:** 4 g + 0.5 g slow i.v. injection every 8 hours;
PYBACTUM, TAZACT, TAZOBID, TAZAR 4 g + 0.5 g per vial inj., also 2 g + 250 mg and 1.0 g + 125 mg vials for inj.

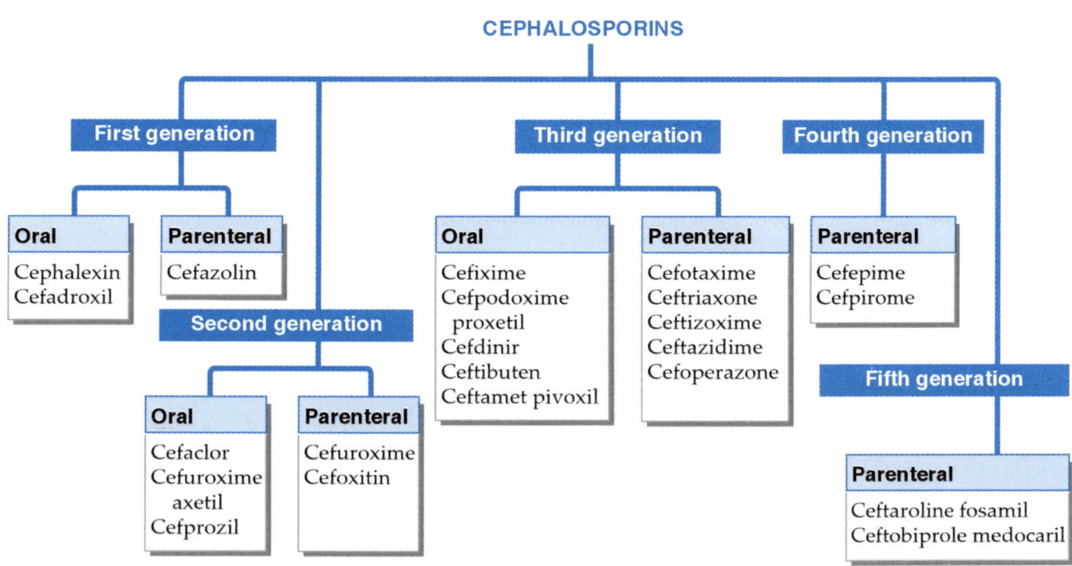
CEPHALOSPORINS
First generation
Oral
Cephalexin
Cefadroxil
Parenteral
Cefazolin
Second generation
Oral
Cefaclor
Cefuroxime axetil
Cefprozil
Parenteral
Cefuroxime
Cefoxitin
Third generation
Oral
Cefixime
Cefpodoxime proxetil
Cefdinir
Ceftibuten
Ceftamet pivoxil
Parenteral
Cefotaxime
Ceftriaxone
Ceftizoxime
Ceftazidime
Cefoperazone
Fourth generation
Parenteral
Cefepime
Cefpirome
Fifth generation
Parenteral
Ceftaroline fosamil
Ceftobiprole medocaril

Preparations

1. **Cefazolin:** 0.5 g 8 hourly (mild cases), 1 g 6 hourly (severe cases), children 25–50 mg/kg/day i.m. or i.v; for surgical prophylaxis 1.0 g half hour before surgery. ORIZOLIN, REFLIN 0.25 g, 0.5 g, 1 g per vial inj.
2. **Cephalexin:** 0.25–1 g 6–8 hourly (children 25–100 mg/kg/day).
   SPORIDEX, ALCEPHIN, CEPHAXIN 250, 500 mg cap, 125 mg/5 ml dry syr., 100 mg/ml pediatric drops.
   ALCEPHIN-LA: Cephalexin + probenecid (250 + 250 mg and 500 + 500 mg) tabs.
3. **Cefadroxil:** 0.5–1 g BD. DROXYL 0.5, 1 g tab, 250 mg/5 ml syr; CEFADROX 0.5 g cap, 125 mg/5 ml syr and 250 mg kid tab; KEFLOXIN 0.5 g cap, 0.25 g distab, 125 mg/5 ml susp.
4. **Cefuroxime:** 0.75 –1.5 g i.m or i.v. 8 hourly, children 30–100 mg/kg/day;
   CEFOGEN, SUPACEF, FUROXIL 250 mg and 750 mg/vial inj.
5. **Cefuroxime axetil:** 250–500 mg BD oral, children half dose;
   CEFTUM, SPIZEF 125, 250, 500 mg captab and 125 mg/5 ml susp.
6. **Cefaclor:** 0.25–1.0 g 8 hourly oral; KEFLOR, VERCEF, DISTACLOR 250 mg cap, 125 and 250 mg distab, 125 mg/5 ml dry syr, 50 mg/ml ped. drops.
7. **Cefprozil:** 250–500 mg BD (20 mg/kg/day); ORPROZIL, ZEMETRIL 250, 500 mg tabs, REFZIL 250 mg, 500 mg tab, 125 mg/5 ml and 250 mg/5 ml syrup.
8. **Cefotaxime:** 1–2 g i.m./i.v. 6–12 hourly (children 50–100 mg/kg/day);
   OMNATAX, ORITAXIM, CLAFORAN 0.25, 0.5, 1.0 g per vial inj.
9. **Ceftizoxime:** 0.5–2 g i.m./i.v. 8 or 12 hourly; CEFIZOX, EPOCELIN 0.5 and 1 g per vial inj.
10. **Ceftriaxone:** Skin/soft tissue/urinary infections: 1–2 g i.v./i.m. per day;
    Meningitis: 4 g followed by 2 g i.v. (children 75–100 mg/kg) once daily for 7–10 days.
    Typhoid: 4 g i.v. daily × 2 days followed by 2 g/day (children 75 mg/kg) till 2 days after fever subsides.

OFRAMAX, MONOCEF, MONOTAX 0.25, 0.5, 1.0 g per vial inj.
Ceftriaxone 250 mg + Sulbactum 125 mg and 1 g + 500 mg: CEFTICHEK, SUPRAXONE vials for inj.
Ceftriaxone 1 g + Tazobactum 125 mg: EXTACEF-TAZO, FINECEF-T, MONTAZ vial for i.m./i.v. inj.

11. **Ceftazidime:** 0.5–2 g i.m. or i.v. every 8 hr, children 30 mg/kg/day. Resistant typhoid 30 mg/kg/day.
FORTUM, CEFAZID, ORZID 0.25, 0.5 and 1 g per vial inj;
COMBITAZ: Ceftazidime 1 g + tazobactam 125 mg/vial inj.
12. **Cefoperazone:** 1–3 g i.m./i.v. 12 hourly; MAGNAMYCIN 0.25 g, 1 g, 2 g inj; CEFOMYCIN, NEGAPLUS 1 g inj.; CEFOBETA, KEFBACTUM, Cefoperazone 500 mg + Sulbactum 500 mg/vial for inj.
13. **Cefixime:** 200–400 mg BD; TOPCEF, ORFIX 100, 200 mg tab/cap, CEFSPAN 100 mg cap, 100 mg/5 ml syr, TAXIM-O 100, 200 mg tab, 50 mg/5ml dry syr.
14. **Cefpodoxime proxetil:** 200 mg BD (max 800 mg/day); CEFOPROX, CEPODEM, DOXCEF 100, 200 mg tab 50 mg/5 ml and 100 mg/5 ml dry syr.
15. **Cefdinir:** 300 mg BD: SEFDIN, ADCEF 300 mg cap, 125 mg/5 ml susp.
16. **Ceftibuten:** 200 mg BD or 400 mg OD; PROCADAX 400 mg cap, 90 mg/5 ml powder for oral suspension.
17. **Ceftamet pivoxil:** 500 mg BD-TDS oral; ALTAMET 250 mg tab, CEPIME-O 500 mg tab.
18. **Cefepime:** 1–2 g (50 mg/kg) i.v. 8–12 hourly; KEFAGE, CEFICAD, CEPIME 0.5, 1.0 g inj.
19. **Cefpirome:** 1–2 g i.m./i.v. 12 hourly; CEFROM, CEFORTH 1.0 g inj., BACIROM, CEFOR 0.25, 0.5, 1.0 g inj.
20. **Ceftaroline fosamil:** 600 mg infused i.v. over 60 min, every 12 hours for 5–14 days;
ZINFORO 600 mg/vial inj.
21. **Ceftobiprole medocaril:** 500 mg infused i.v. over 2 hours every 8 hours.
ZEVTERA 667 mg (equaivalent to ceftobiprole 500 mg) vial powder for reconstitution and i.v. infusion.

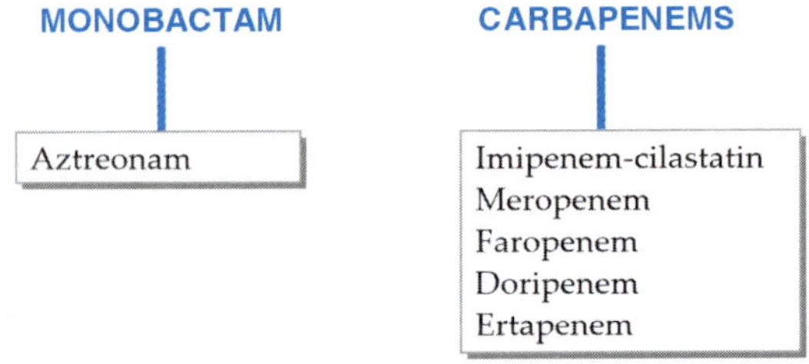

Preparations

1. **Aztreonam:** 0.5–2 g i.m. or i.v. 6–12 hourly; AZENAM 0.5, 1.0, 2.0 g per vial inj.
2. **Imipenem-cilastatin:** 0.5 g i.v. 6 hourly (max 4 g/day). IMINEM 250 + 250 mg and 500 + 500 mg/vial inj., LASTINEM 125 + 125 mg, 250 + 250 mg, 500 + 500 mg and 1 g + 1 g per vial inj.
3. **Meropenem:** 0.5–2 g i.v. (10–40 mg/kg) 8 hourly; MENEM, MERONEM, MICROPENAM 0.5, 1.0 g per vial inj.
4. **Faropenem:** 150–300 mg TDS oral; FARONEM, FAROZET 150, 200 mg tab.
5. **Doripenem:** 500 mg slow i.v. infusion over 1 hour every 8 hours; DORIGLEN, DORICRIT 500 mg/vial inj., SUDOPEN 250, 500 mg/vial inj.
6. **Ertapenem:** 1 g infused i.v. over 60 min daily for 7–14 days; ERTACRIT, ZIVATOR 1.0 g/vial inj (to be reconstituted).

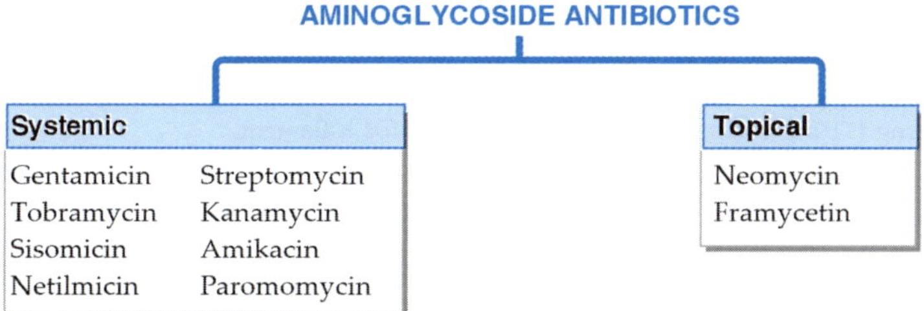

Preparations

1. **Gentamicin:** 3–5 mg/kg/day i.m. in a single dose or divided in 8 hourly doses or in an i.v. line over 30–60 min (dose reduction needed in elderly and in renal insufficiency), 0.1–0.3% topically in eye or on skin. GARAMYCIN, GENTASPORIN, GENTICYN 20, 60, 80, 240 mg per vial inj; also 0.3% eye/ear drops, 0.1% skin cream.
2. **Tobramycin:** 3–5 mg/kg/day i.m. or i.v. infusion in 1–3 doses; TOBACIN 20, 60, 80 mg in 2 ml inj. 0.3% eye drops. TOBRANEG 20, 40, 80 mg per 2 ml inj., TOBRABACT 0.3% eye drops.
3. **Netilmicin:** 4–6 mg/kg/day i.m. in 1–3 doses; NETROMYCIN 10, 25, 50 mg in 1 ml, 200 mg in 2 ml and 300 mg in 3 ml inj., NETICIN 200 mg (2 ml), 300 mg (3 ml) inj.
4. **Streptomycin:** Acute infections: 1 g (0.75 g in those above 50 yr age) i.m. (15 mg/kg) BD for 7–10 days.

   Tuberculosis: 1 g (elderly 0.75 g) i.m. OD for 60 days;
   AMBISTRYN–S 0.75 g, 1 g dry powder per vial for inj.
5. **Kanamycin:** 0.5 g i.m. BD (15 mg/kg/day): KANCIN, KANAMAC 0.5, 1 g inj.

6. **Amikacin:** 15 mg/kg/day i.m. in 1–3 doses; urinary tract infection 7.5 mg/kg/day;
   AMICIN, MIKACIN, MIKAJECT 250 mg, 500 mg in 2 ml inj.
7. **Paromomycin:** *Oral*: 500 mg TDS (25–30 mg/kg/day) for amoebiasis, giardiasis, etc.
   Intramuscular: 15 mg (11 mg base) per kg/day for 21 days for Kala-azar.
8. **Neomycin:** 0.25–1 g QID oral, 0.3–0.5% topical.
   NEOMYCIN SULPHATE 350, 500 mg tab, 0.3% skin oint, 0.5% skin cream, eye oint.
   NEBASULF: Neomycin sulph. 5 mg, bacitracin 250 U, sulfacetamide 60 mg/g oint. and powder for surface application.
   NEOSPORIN: Neomycin 3400 iu, polymyxin B 5000 iu, bacitracin 400 iu/g oint; NEOSPORIN-H: Neomycin 3400 iu, polymyxin B 10000 iu, hydrocortisone 10 mg per ml ear drops.
9. **Framycetin:** 0.5%–1.0% topically in eye or on skin;
   SOFRAMYCIN 1% skin cream, 0.5% eye drops or oint.

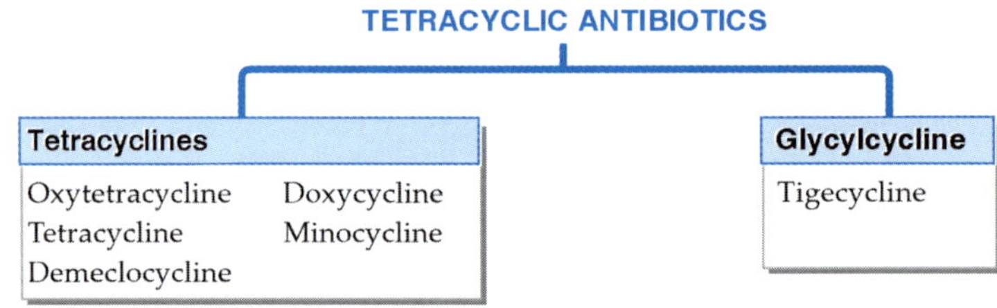

1. **Oxytetracycline:** 250–500 mg TDS–QID oral, 500 mg 6–12 hourly by slow i.v. inj; 1–3% by topical application; TERRAMYCIN 250, 500 mg cap, 50 mg/ml in 10 ml vials inj; 3% skin oint, 1% eye/ear oint.
2. **Tetracycline:** 250–500 mg TDS–QID oral; 1–3% topically in eye/ear/on skin; ACHROMYCIN, HOSTACYCLINE, RESTECLIN 250, 500 mg cap, 3% skin oint, 1% eye/ear drops and oint.
3. **Demeclocycline (Demethylchlortetracycline):** 300–600 mg BD oral; LEDERMYCIN 150, 300 mg cap/tab.
4. **Doxycycline:** 200 mg initially followed by 100–200 mg OD oral; TETRADOX, DOXICIP, DOXT, NOVADOX 100 mg cap.
5. **Minocycline:** 100 mg OD–BD oral; CYANOMYCIN, MINOZ, DIVAINE 50, 100 mg caps.
6. **Tigecycline:** 100 mg loading dose, followed by 50 mg 12 hourly i.v. infusion over 30–60 min for 5–14 days. TYGACIL, TEVRAN, TIGIMAX 50 mg lyophilized powder per vial inj.

Chloramphenicol

1. **Chloramphenicol:** 250–500 mg 6 hourly oral (max 28 g total in a course), children 25–50 mg/kg/day; 0.5–1% topically in eye, 5–10% topically in ear; rarely 1% on skin; CHLOROMYCETIN, ENTEROMYCETIN, PARAXIN, 250 mg, 500 mg cap, 1% eye oint, 0.5% eye drops, 5% ear drops, 1% applicaps, VANMYCETIN 0.4% eye drops, 250 mg opticaps.
2. **Chloramphenicol palmitate** (tasteless insoluble ester of chloramphenicol for liquid oral formulation): CHLOROMYCETIN PALMITATE, ENTEROMYCETIN, PARAXIN 125 mg/5 ml oral susp.
3. **Chloramphenicol succinate** (soluble ester of chloramphenicol for i.v. injection): ENTEROMYCETIN, CHLOROMYCETIN SUCCINATE, PARAXIN 1 g/vial inj.

Macrolide Antibiotics

1. Erythromycin: 250–500 mg 6 hourly (max. 4 g/day), children 30–60 mg/kg/day.
   (a) Erythromycin (base): EROMED 333 mg tab, 125 mg/5 ml susp.
   (b) Erythromycin stearate: ERYTHROCIN 250, 500 mg tabs, 100 mg/5 ml susp., 100 mg/ml ped. drops. ERYSTER 250 mg tab, 100 mg/5 ml dry syr.
   (c) Erythromycin estolate (lauryl sulfate): ALTHROCIN 250, 500 mg tab, 125 mg kid tab, 125 mg/5 ml and 250 mg/5 ml dry syr, 100 mg/ml ped. drops, E-MYCIN 100, 250 mg tab, 100 mg/5 ml dry syr; EMTHROCIN 250 mg tab, 125 mg/5 ml dry syr.
   (d) Erythromycin ethylsuccinate: ERYTHROCIN 500 mg tab, 100 mg/ml drops, 125 mg/5 ml syr.
2. Roxithromycin: 150–300 mg BD 30 min before meals, children 2.5–5 mg/kg BD; ROXID, ROXIBID, RULIDE 150, 300 mg tab, 50 mg kid tab, 50 mg/5 ml liquid; ROXEM 50 mg kid tab, 150 mg tab.
3. Clarithromycin: 250 mg BD for 7 days; severe cases 500 mg BD upto 14 days; CLARIBID 250, 500 mg tab, 250 mg/5 ml dry syr; CLARIMAC 250, 500 mg tabs; SYNCLAR 250 mg tab, 125 mg/5 ml dry syr.
4. Azithromycin: 500 mg once daily 1 hour before or 2 hours after food (children above 6 month 10 mg/kg) for 3 days is sufficient for most upper respiratory infections; AZITHRAL 250, 500 mg cap and 250 mg per 5 ml dry syr; AZIWOK 250 mg cap, 100 mg kid tab, 100 mg/5 ml and 200 mg/5 ml susp. AZEE 250 mg, 500 mg tab. AZIWIN 100, 250, 500 mg tab, 200 mg/5 ml liq. Also AZITHRAL 500 mg inj. for i.m. use.
5. Spiramycin: 3 million units (MU) twice daily oral; ROVAMYCIN 1.5 MU, 3 MU tabs, 0.375 MU/5 ml susp.

Lincosamide Antibiotics

1. **Clindamycin:** 150–300 mg (Children 3–6 mg/kg) QID oral; 200–600 mg i.v. 8 hourly; DALCAP 150 mg cap; CLINCIN 150, 300 mg cap; DALCIN, DALCINEX 150, 300 mg cap, 300 mg/2 ml and 600 mg/4 ml inj. ACNESOL, CLINDAC-A 1% topical solution and gel for acne vulgaris.
2. **Lincomycin:** 500 mg TDS–QID oral; 600 mg i.m. or by i.v. infusion 6–12 hrly; LINCOCIN 500 mg cap, 600 mg/2 ml inj; LYNX 250, 500 mg cap, 125 mg/5 ml syr, 300 mg/ml inj in 1, 2 ml amp.

Aminocyclitol Antibiotic

1. **Spectinomycin:** Gonorrhoea—2 g i.m. single dose (4 g in resistant cases); disseminated gonococcal infection—2 g i.m. BD.
   SPECTIN, TROBICIN 2 g vial for i.m. inj.

Glycopeptide Antibiotics

1. **Vancomycin:** 125–500 mg oral (for pseudomembranous enterocolitis), 0.5 g 6 hourly or 1.0 g 12 hourly by i.v. infusion over 1 hour;
   VANCOCIN-CP; VANCOGEN, VANCORID-CP 500 mg/vial inj;
   VANCOLED 0.5, 1.0 g inj, VANCOMYCIN 500 mg tab, VANLID 250 mg cap, 0.5 g/vial and 1 g/vial inj.
2. **Teicoplanin:** 400 mg first day—then 200 mg daily i.v. or i.m.; severe infection 400 mg 12 hourly × 3 doses—then 400 mg daily; TARGOCID, TECOPLAN, TECONIN 200, 400 mg per vial inj. for reconstitution.

Oxazolidinones

1. **Linezolid:** 600 mg BD, oral/i.v.;
   LIZOLID 600 mg tab; LINOX, LINOSPAN 600 mg tab, 600 mg/300 ml i.v. infusion.
2. **Tedizolid:** 200 mg once daily oral or by slow i.v. infusion.

Streptogramins

1. **Quinupristin/Dalfopristin (30:70):** 7.5 mg/kg infused i.v. over 60 min every 8–12 hours;
   SYNERCID: Quinupristin 150 mg + Dalfopristin 350 mg per vial inj.

Lipopeptide Antibiotic

1. **Daptomycin:** 4 mg/kg (for skin and soft tissue infection), 6 mg/kg (for bacteraemia/endocarditis) i.v. once daily.
   DAPTOCURE 350 mg/vial for reconstitution before injection.

Polypeptide Antibiotics

1. **Polymyxin B:** 5000–10,000 U/g for topical application (1 mg = 10,000 U);
   NEOSPORIN POWDER: 5000 U with neomycin sulf. 3400 U and bacitracin 400 U per g.
   NEOSPORIN EYE DROPS: 5000 U with neomycin sulf. 1700 U and gramicidin 0.25 mg per ml.
   NEOSPORIN-H EAR DROPS: 10,000 U with neomycin sulf. 3400 U and hydrocortisone 10 mg per ml.
2. **Colistin sulfate:** 25–100 mg TDS oral; WALAMYCIN 12.5 mg (25000 i.u.) per 5 ml dry syr, COLISTOP 12.5 mg/5 ml and 25 mg/5 ml dry syr.
3. **Bacitracin:** 250–500 U/g for topical application (1 U = 26 μg); In NEBASULF: bacitracin 250 U + neomycin 5 mg + sulfacetamide 60 mg/g powder, skin oint, eye oint; in NEOSPORIN 400 U/g powder.

Urinary Antiseptics

1. **Nitrofurantoin:** 50–100 mg 3 times a day oral for treatment of urinary tract infection; 100 mg at bed time daily for long term suppressive treatment of lower urinary tract infection.

   FURADANTIN, URIFAST 50, 100 mg tab, URINIF, NIFTRAN; 100 mg tab.
   NEPHROGESIC: Nitrofurantion 50 mg + phenazopyridine 100 mg tab.

2. **Fosfomycin:** 3 g single oral dose for uncomplicated lower urinary tract infection in women; 3 g oral every 3rd day for 9–21 days for prostatitis in males.
   FOSFOCIN, NOVEFOS, FOSFOGEN 3 g powder in sachet for dissolving in water before taking.
3. **Methenamine (Hexamine) mandelate:** 1.0 g 3–4 times/day oral; MANDELAMINE 0.5 g, 1.0 g tabs.
4. **Nalidixic acid:** 0.5–1 g TDS–QID oral (*See* p. 145)

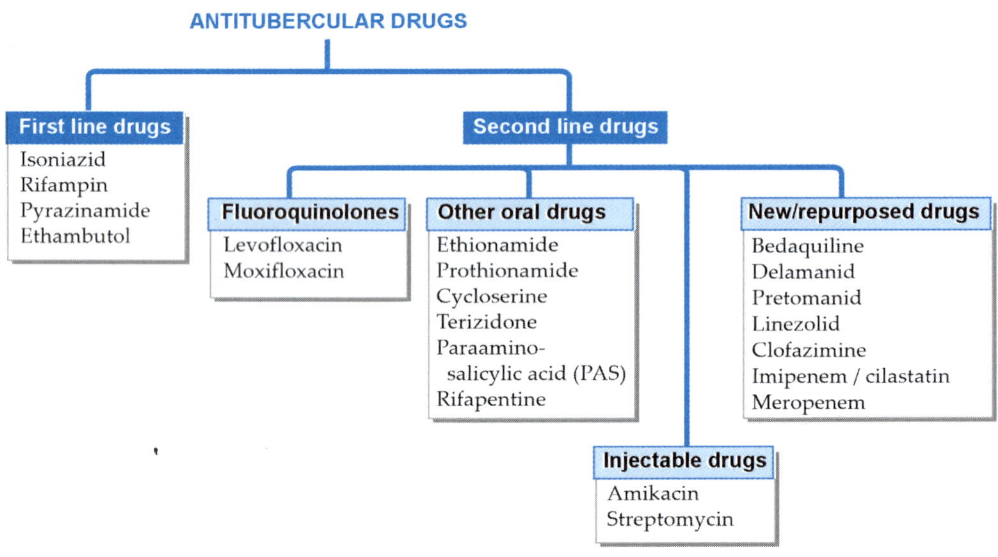
ANTITUBERCULAR DRUGS
First line drugs
Isoniazid
Rifampin
Pyrazinamide
Ethambutol
Second line drugs
Fluoroquinolones
Levofloxacin
Moxifloxacin
Other oral drugs
Ethionamide
Prothionamide
Cycloserine
Terizidone
Paraamino-
salicylic acid (PAS)
Rifapentine
Injectable drugs
Amikacin
Streptomycin
New/repurposed drugs
Bedaquiline
Delamanid
Pretomanid
Linezolid
Clofazimine
Imipenem / cilastatin
Meropenem

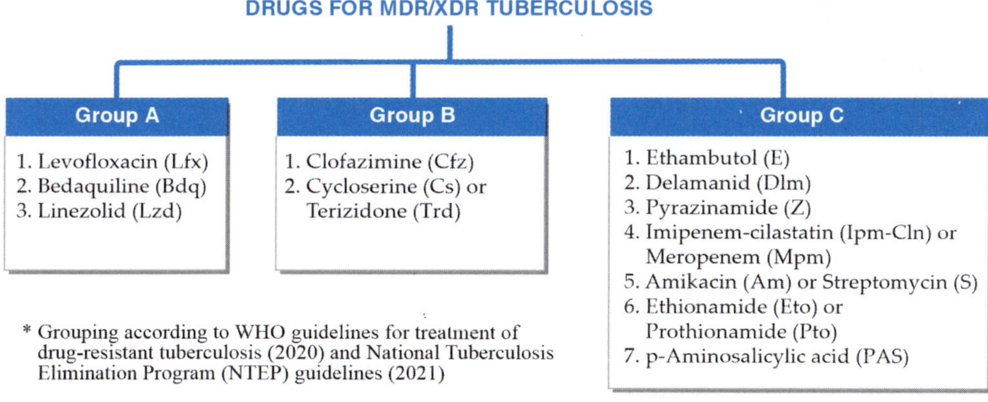

* Grouping according to WHO guidelines for treatment of drug-resistant tuberculosis (2020) and National Tuberculosis Elimination Program (NTEP) guidelines (2021)

Preparations

Antitubercular Drugs

1. **Isoniazid (Isonicotinic acid hydrazide, INH):** 5 mg/kg daily oral; ISONEX 100, 300 mg tabs, ISOKIN 100 mg tab, 100 mg per 5 ml liq.
2. **Rifampin (Rifampicin):** 600 mg (10 mg/kg) daily oral one hour before or two hours after meals; RCIN 150, 300, 450, 600 mg caps, 100 mg/5 ml susp. RIMACTANE, RIMPIN 150, 300, 450 mg caps, 100 mg/5 ml syr; RIFAMYCIN 450 mg cap, ZUCOX 300, 450, 600 mg tabs.

3. **Pyrazinamide:** 25 mg/kg daily oral;
PYZINA 0.5, 0.75, 1.0 g tabs, 0.3 g kid tab; PZA-CIBA 0.5, 0.75 g tabs, 250 mg/5 ml syr; RIZAP 0.75, 1.0 g tabs.
4. **Ethambutol:** 15 mg/kg daily oral; MYCOBUTOL, MYAMBUTOL, COMBUTOL 0.2, 0.4, 0.6, 0.8, 1.0 g tabs.
5. **Streptomycin:** 1000 mg (15 mg/kg) daily i.m.; patients over 60 years age—reduce dose to 10 mg/kg or 500–750 mg/day i.m. AMBISTRYN-S 0.75 g and 1.0 g dry powder per vial for i.m. inj after reconstitution.
6. **Paraaminosalicylic acid (PAS):** 10–12 g (200 mg/kg) per day oral in divided doses;
SODIUM-PAS 0.5 g tab, 80 g/100 g granules.
7. **Ethionamide:** 0.5–0.75 g (10–15 mg/kg) per day oral; ETHIDE, ETHIOKOX, MYOBID 250 mg tab.
8. **Prothionamide:** 0.5–0.75 g (10–15 mg/kg/day) oral; PROTHICID, PETHIDE 250 mg tab.
9. **Cycloserine:** 250 mg BD, increased if tolerated upto 750 mg per day oral;
CYCLORIN, COXERIN, MYSER 250 mg cap.
10. **Terizidone:** 500–750 mg/day oral; TERICOX 250 mg cap.
11. **Amikacin:** 0.75–1.0 g (15 mg/kg) i.m. daily; AMICIN, MIKACIN, MIKAJECT 250 mg, 500 mg inj.
12. **Levofloxacin:** 1000 mg OD (for body weight >45 kg), 750 mg (for BW 30–45 kg), 250 mg (for BW 16–29 kg).
13. **Moxifloxacin:** 400 mg OD (for body weight >30 kg), 200 mg (for BW 16–29 kg).
14. **Rifapentine:** 600 mg once or twice a week during the continuation phase as substitute for daily rifampin.
15. **Bedaquiline:** 400 mg/day for 2 weeks followed by 200 mg 3 times a week for the next 22 weeks.
16. **Delamanid:** 100 mg twice daily (for age ≥ 12 years), 50 mg twice daily (for age 6–11 years) for 24 weeks.
17. **Pretomanid:** 200 mg/day for 26 weeks.
18. **Linezolid:** 600 mg/day (for BW >30 kg), 300 mg/day (for BW 16–29 kg).
19. **Clofazimine:** 200 mg/day (for BW >70 kg), 100 mg/day (for BW 30–69 kg), 50 mg/day (for BW 16–29 kg).

20. **Imipenem-cilastatin:** 2 g twice daily.
21. **Meropenem:** 1 g thrice daily.

Some antitubercular combinations

RIFATER: Rifampin 120 mg, isoniazid 80 mg, pyrazinamide 250 mg tab.

R-CINEX: Rifampin 600 mg, isoniazid 300 mg tab; R-CINEX-Z: Rifampin 225 mg, isoniazid 150 mg, pyrazinamide 750 mg tab. RIMACTAZID, RIFADIN-INH, Rifampin 450 mg, isoniazid 300 mg tab.

MYCONEX 600 and 800; Isoniazid 300 mg, ethambutol 600 mg or 800 mg tab, COMBUNEX Isoniazid 300 mg, ethambutol 800 mg tab.

ARZIDE, ISORIFAM: Rifampin 450 mg, isoniazid 300 mg cap.

INABUTOL: Isoniazid 150 mg, ethambutol 400 mg tab; INABUTOL FORTE—double strength.

ISOKIN–300: Isoniazid 300 mg, vit B_6 10 mg tab.

IPCAZIDE: Isoniazid 100 mg, vit B_6 5 mg per 5 ml liq.

Antitubercular Combipacks (packs of 1 day's dose)

AKT-4: R 450 mg 1 cap + Z 750 mg 2 tab + E 800 mg + H 300 mg 1 tab.
AKT-3: R 450 mg 1 cap + E 800 mg + H 300 mg 1 tab.
CX-5: R 450 mg 1 cap + Z 750 mg 2 tab + E 800 mg + H 300 mg + pyridoxine 10 mg 1 tab.
RIFACOM-Z and RIMACTAZID-Z: R 450 mg + H 300 mg 1 tab. + Z 750 mg 2 tab.
RIFACOM-EZ: R 450 mg + H 300 mg 1 tab. + Z 750 mg 2 tab + E 800 mg 1 tab.

Note: *See* Index for preparations of ciprofloxacin, ofloxacin, levofloxacin and moxifloxacin.

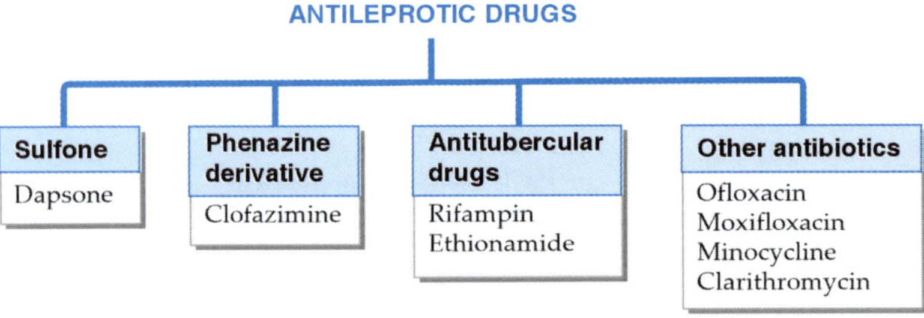

Antileprotic Drugs

1. Dapsone (Diaminodiphenyl sulfone, DDS): 100 mg/day; DAPSONE 25, 50, 100 mg tab.
2. Clofazimine: 50 mg daily + 300 mg once a month; CLOFOZINE, HANSEPRAN 50, 100 mg caps.
3. Rifampin: 600 mg once a month
4. Ethionamide: 250 mg/day oral
5. Ofloxacin: 400 mg/day oral
6. Moxifloxacin: 400 mg/day oral
7. Minocycline: 100 mg/day oral
8. Clarithromycin: 500 mg/day oral.

Note: See Index for preparations of other drugs.

For erythema nodosum leprosum (type 2)

Thalidomide: 100–300 mg OD at bed time; THAANGIO 100 mg cap., THALODA 50, 100 mg cap. (For multiple myeloma—200 mg OD; max 800 mg/day).

Antifungal, Antiviral, Antiprotozoal and Anthelmintic Drugs

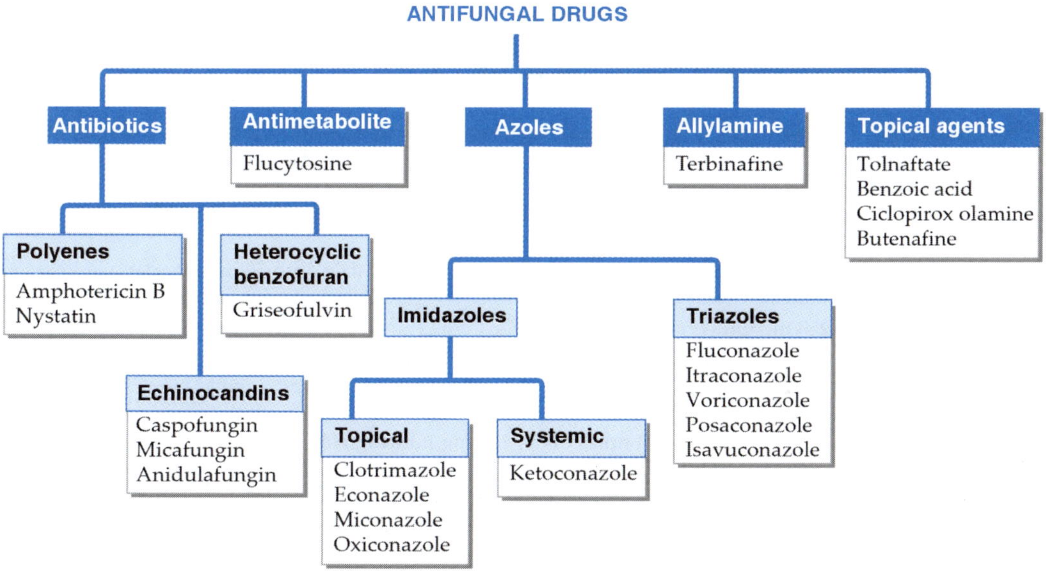

ANTIFUNGAL DRUGS

- **Antibiotics**
  - **Polyenes**
    - Amphotericin B
    - Nystatin
  - **Echinocandins**
    - Caspofungin
    - Micafungin
    - Anidulafungin
  - **Heterocyclic benzofuran**
    - Griseofulvin
- **Antimetabolite**
  - Flucytosine
- **Azoles**
  - **Imidazoles**
    - **Topical**
      - Clotrimazole
      - Econazole
      - Miconazole
      - Oxiconazole
    - **Systemic**
      - Ketoconazole
  - **Triazoles**
    - Fluconazole
    - Itraconazole
    - Voriconazole
    - Posaconazole
    - Isavuconazole
- **Allylamine**
  - Terbinafine
- **Topical agents**
  - Tolnaftate
  - Benzoic acid
  - Ciclopirox olamine
  - Butenafine

Preparations

1. **Amphotericin B (deoxycholate):** 0.3–0.7 mg/kg daily by slow i.v. infusion over 4–8 hours (total dose 3–4 g); 0.5 mg intrathecal, 3% topically in ear, 50–100 mg QID oral; FUNGIZONE INTRAVENOUS, MYCOL 50 mg dry powder per vial for i.v. infusion, FUNGIZONE OTIC 3% ear drops.
   Liposomal amphotericin B: 3-5 mg/kg/day i.v. infusion;
   FUNGISOME 10 mg, 25 mg, 50 mg per vial inj, AMPHOLIP 10 mg/2 ml, 50 mg/10 ml, 100 mg/20 ml inj.
2. **Nystatin:** 5 lac U 8 hourly oral, 1 lac U vaginal insertion every night, 10,000 U/ml for buccal application; 1 lac U per g for application over skin.
   MYCOSTATIN 5 lac U tab, 1 lac U vaginal tab, 1 lac U/g oint.
3. **Caspofungin:** 70 mg infused i.v. over 1 hour (loading dose), followed by 50 mg i.v. daily.
   CANCIDAS, CASPOGIN 70 mg in 10 ml and 50 mg in 10 ml inj.
4. **Micafungin:** 100–150 mg i.v./day, children 3 mg/kg/day; prophylactic dose 50 mg i.v./day.
   MICAFUNG PLUS 50 mg, 100 mg/vial inj., MICONA-IV, MICANFA 50 mg/vial for inj.
5. **Griseofulvin:** 125–250 mg QID oral taken with meals; GRISOVIN–FP, GRISORAL, WALAVIN 250 mg tab.
6. **Clotrimazole:** 1% topical application twice daily, 100 mg intravaginal at bed time:
   SURFAZ, 1% lotion, cream, powder; 1% ear drop with 2% lidocaine; 100 mg vaginal tab. CANDID 1% cream, mouth paint, powder, 1% ear drops with 2% lidocaine.
7. **Econazole:** 1% topical application 2–3 times daily, 150 mg intravaginal every night;
   ECANOL VAGINAL 150 mg vaginal tab.
8. **Miconazole:** 2% topical application 2–3 times daily, 100 mg intravaginal nightly;
   DAKTARIN 2% gel, 2% powder and solution; GYNODAKTARIN 2% vaginal gel; ZOLE 2% oint, lotion, dusting powder and spray, 1% ear drops, 100 mg vaginal ovules.

9. **Oxiconazole:** 1% topical;
ZODERM-E oxiconazole 1% + benzoic acid 0.2% cream and lotion; AUXERG 1% cream.
10. **Ketoconazole:** 200 mg OD oral, 2% topical application;
FUNGICIDE, NIZRAL, KETOVATE 200 mg tab, FUNGINOC, NIZRAL 2% oint, 2% shampoo (for dandruff), KETOVATE 2% cream, DANRUF 2% shampoo, HYPHORAL 2% lotion.
11. **Fluconazole:** For tinea infections, cutaneous and vaginal candidiasis 150 mg oral weekly for 4 weeks; for candida esophagitis 100 mg/day for 2–3 weeks, for systemic mycosis 200–400 mg daily oral/i.v. for 4–12 weeks;
SYSCAN, ZOCON, FORCAN, FLUZON 50, 100, 150, 200 mg caps, 200 mg/100 ml i.v. infusion.
12. **Itraconazole:** 200 mg OD–BD oral or i.v. (for systemic mycosis), 200 mg OD oral for vaginal candidiasis and dermatophytosis, 200 mg/day for 3 months to treat onychomycosis;
SPORANOX, CANDITRAL 100 mg cap, ITASPOR 100 mg cap, 200 mg/20 ml vial for i.v. injection.
13. **Voriconazole:** Oral–200 mg BD taken 1 hour before or 1 hour after meal; Intravenous—initially 6 mg/kg 12 hourly 2 doses, then 3–4 mg/kg 12 hourly. The drug is to be reconstituted and diluted, infused at not more than 3 mg/kg/hr.
VFEND 50 mg, 200 mg tabs, 40 mg/ml oral susp; 200 mg vial for i.v. infusion; FUNGIVOR 200 mg tab.
14. **Posaconazole:** 200 mg 4 times a day or 400 mg twice a day with meals. NOXAFIL 200 mg/5 ml susp.
15. **Terbinafine:** 250 mg OD oral, 1% topical application twice daily; LAMISIL, SEBIFIN, DASKIL 250 mg tab, 1% topical cream. EXIFINE 125, 250 mg tabs, 1% cream, TERBIDERM 1% cream.
16. **Tolnaftate:** 1% topical application; TINADERM, TINAVATE 1% lotion, TOLNADERM 1% cream.
17. **Ciclopirox olamine:** 1% topical and vaginal application;
BATRAFEN 1% cream, 1% topical solution, 1% vaginal cream, OLAMIN 1% cream, ONYLAC NAIL LACQUER 8% nail lacquer.

18. **Benzoic acid:** 5% topical application; RINGCUTTER, WHITEFIELDS OINTMENT 5% benzoic acid + 3% salicylic acid oint/cream.
19. **Butenafine:** 1% topical; BUTOP, FINTOP 1% cream.

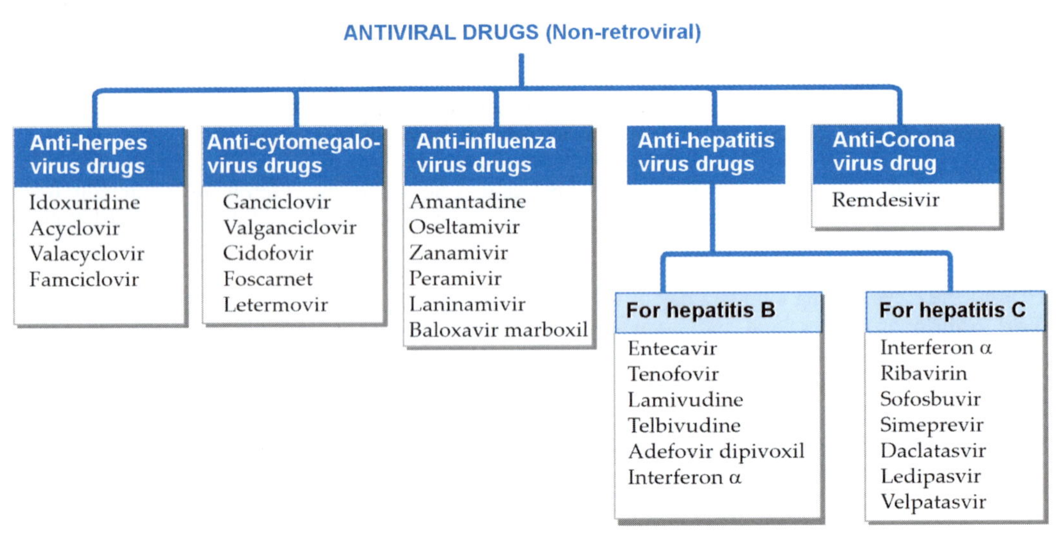

Preparations

1. **Idoxuridine:** 0.1% topically in eye 1 hourly to 4 hourly, apply 0.1% eye ointment at night; IDURIN, TOXIL 0.1% eye drops and oint.
2. **Acyclovir:** 400 mg 5 times a day oral; 5 mg/kg 8 hourly by slow i.v. infusion, 5% topical application 6 times a day; ZOVIRAX 200, 800 mg tab, 250 mg/vial for i.v. inj; CYCLOVIR 200 mg tab, 5% skin cream; HERPEX 200 mg tab, 3% eye oint, 5% skin cream; OCUVIR 200, 400, 800 mg tab, 3% eye oint, ACIVIR-DT 200, 400, 800 mg tab. ACIVIR EYE 3% oint.
3. **Valacyclovir:** For genital herpes simplex 1.0 g BD × 10 days, suppressive treatment 0.5 g OD × 6–12 months. For orolabial herpes 2 g BD × 1 day; For herpes zoster 1 g TDS × 7 days.
   VALCIVIR 0.5 g, 1.0 g tabs.
4. **Famciclovir:** Genital herpes (1st episode) 250 mg TDS × 5 days; recurrent cases 250 mg BD for upto 1 year. Herpes zoster and orolabial herpes 500 mg TDS for 7–10 days. FAMTREX 250, 500 mg tabs.
5. **Ganciclovir:** For treatment and prophylaxis of CMV infections—5 mg/kg BD initially, followed by once daily; GANGUARD 250, 500 mg cap, 500 mg/vial powder for inj.
6. **Valganciclovir:** 900 mg OD or BD oral; VALGAN, VALSTEAD 450 mg tab.
7. **Cidofovir:** 5 mg/kg i.v. weekly and then fortmightly; CIDNAVIR, CIDOFOVIR 75 mg/ml inj in 5 ml vial.
8. **Foscarnet:** 40–60 mg/kg infused i.v. every 8 hours for 2–3 weeks, followed by 60–120 mg/kg/i.v. daily; FOSCAVIR 6 g/250 ml inj.
9. **Amantadine:** Prophylactic 100 mg OD, therapeutic 100 mg BD for 5 days; elderly—half dose, children 5 mg/kg/day; AMANTREL 100 mg tab.
10. **Oseltamivir:** therapeutic dose—75 mg BD × 5 days; prophylactic dose—75 mg OD;
    TAMIFLU, ANTIFLU 75 mg cap, 12 mg/ml susp, FLUVIR 75 mg cap.

11. **Zanamivir:** therapeutic dose—10 mg BD; prophylactic dose—10 mg OD; through breath actuated inhaler or rotacaps; VIRENZA 5 mg per actuation powder inhaler rotacaps, Z-FLU 5 mg dry powder inhaler cap.
12. **Peramivir:** 600 mg (single dose) to be diluted and injected i.v. over 15–20 min within 48 hours of influenza symptom onset.
    RAPIVAB 200 mg/vial inj. (3 vials to be used for treating influenza in adults).
13. **Lamivudine:** 100 mg OD for chronic hepatitis B;
    LAMIVIR-HBV 100 mg tab; LAMIDAC, VIROLAM, LAMUVID 100, 150 mg tabs.
14. **Entecavir:** 0.5 mg OD; for lamivudine resistant HBV 1 mg OD; ENTAVIR 0.5 mg, 1.0 mg tabs.
15. **Adefovir dipivoxil:** 10 mg/day oral; ADESERA, ADFOVIR 10 mg tab.
16. **Tenofovir disoproxil fumarate:** 300 mg OD; TENOF, TENTIDE, TENVIR 300 mg tab.
17. **Telbivudine:** 600 mg OD; SEBIVO 600 mg tab.
18. **Ribavirin:** 200 mg QID (children 15 mg/kg/day); VIRAZIDE, RIBAVIN 100, 200 mg caps, 50 mg/5 ml syr.
19. **Interferon α_{2A}:** 2.5–5 MU/m^2 s.c. or i.m. 3 times per week; ALFERON 3MU/vial inj.
20. **Interferon α_{2B}:** 3–10 MU s.c. or i.m. thrice weekly;
    REALFA-2B, SHANFERON, VIRAFERON 3MU, 5MU vials for inj.
21. **Peginterferon α_{2A}:** 180 μg/week s.c.; PEGASYS 135 μg/vial and 180 μg/vial inj.; EXKURA 180 μg in 0.5 ml inj.
22. **Peginterferon α_{2B}:** PEGIHEP 80 μg, 100 μg and 120 μg single dose vial.
23. **Sofosbuvir:** 400 mg daily with meals; MYHEP, SOFOCURE, HEPCINAT, SOVIHEP 400 mg tab.
24. **Simeprevir:** 150 mg per day; OLYSIO, GALEXOS 150 mg cap.
25. **Daclatasvir:** 60 mg/day, reduce dose to 30 mg/day in patients receiving CYP3A inhibitors, and increase to 90 mg/day in those on CYP3A inducers; HEPEDAC, DACIHEP, MYDEKLA 60 mg tab.

25. **Ledipasvir:** 90 mg per day along with sofosbuvir 400 mg;
SOFAB-LP, HEPCINAT-LP: ledipasvir 90 mg + sofosbuvir 400 mg tab.
26. **Velpatasvir:** 100 mg/day along with sofosbuvir 400 mg/day;
VELPANAT: velpatasvir 100 mg + sofosbuvir 400 mg tab.
27. **Remdesivir:** Initially 200 mg i.v., followed by 100 mg once daily i.v. for upto 5 days;
CIPREMI: 100 mg/vial inj.

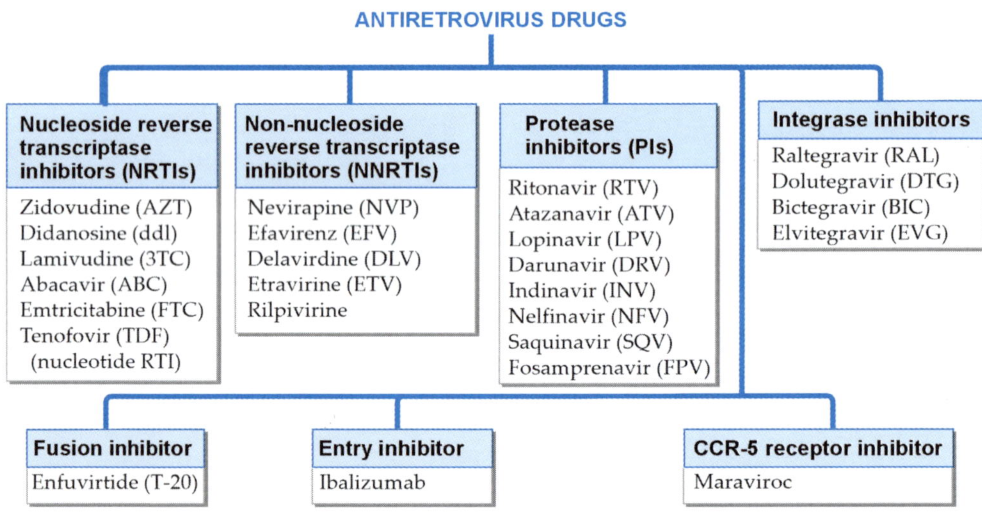
ANTIRETROVIRUS DRUGS
Nucleoside reverse transcriptase inhibitors (NRTIs)
Zidovudine (AZT)
Didanosine (ddl)
Lamivudine (3TC)
Abacavir (ABC)
Emtricitabine (FTC)
Tenofovir (TDF) (nucleotide RTI)
Non-nucleoside reverse transcriptase inhibitors (NNRTIs)
Nevirapine (NVP)
Efavirenz (EFV)
Delavirdine (DLV)
Etravirine (ETV)
Rilpivirine
Protease inhibitors (PIs)
Ritonavir (RTV)
Atazanavir (ATV)
Lopinavir (LPV)
Darunavir (DRV)
Indinavir (INV)
Nelfinavir (NFV)
Saquinavir (SQV)
Fosamprenavir (FPV)
Integrase inhibitors
Raltegravir (RAL)
Dolutegravir (DTG)
Bictegravir (BIC)
Elvitegravir (EVG)
Fusion inhibitor
Enfuvirtide (T-20)
Entry inhibitor
Ibalizumab
CCR-5 receptor inhibitor
Maraviroc

Preparations

1. **Zidovudine (Azidothymidine, AZT):** Adults 300 mg BD; Children 180 mg/m^2 (max 200 mg) BD.
   RETROVIR, ZIDOVIR 100 mg cap 300 mg tab, 50 mg/5 ml syr, ZIDOMAX, ZYDOWIN 100 mg cap, 300 mg tab (to be taken with plenty of water).
2. **Didanosine:** 400 mg/day (for ≥ 60 kg BW), 250 mg/day (< 50 kg BW); 1 hour before or 2 hours after meals; DINEX EC, DD RETRO, VIROSINE DR 250, 400 mg tabs.
3. **Lamivudine:** *For HIV infection*—150 mg BD or 300 mg OD;
   LAMIVIR 150 mg tab, 150 mg/5 ml soln; HEPTAVIR, LAMIDAC, LAMUVID 100, 150 mg tabs.
4. **Abacavir:** 300 mg BD or 600 mg OD; ABAMUNE, ABAVIR 300 mg tab.
5. **Tenofovir disoproxil fumarate:** 300 mg OD; TENVIR-L: tenofovir 300 mg + lamivudine 300 mg tab. TRIO-DAY: tenofovir 300 mg + lamivudine 300 mg + efavirenz 600 mg tab.
6. **Emtricitabine:** 200 mg OD; TENVIR-EM, TENOF-EM, TAVIN-EM: emtricitabine 200 mg + tenofovir 300 mg tab; VIRADAY, TRUSTIVA, VONAVIR: emtricitabine 200 mg + tenofovir 300 mg + efavirenz 600 mg tab.
7. **Nevirapine:** 200 mg/day oral to be increased after 2 weeks to 200 mg BD;
   NEVIMUNE, NEVIVIR, NEVIPAN, NEVIRETRO 200 mg tab.
8. **Efavirenz:** 600 mg OD on empty stomach; EFFERVEN, VIRANZ, EVIRENZ, 200 mg cap, 600 mg tab.
9. **Etravirine:** 200 mg BD after meals; INTRAVIR 200 mg tab.
10. **Atazanavir:** 300 mg OD with ritonavir 100 mg taken at meal time; ATAZOR 100, 150, 200, 300 mg caps.
11. **Indinavir:** 800 mg TDS; INDIVAN, INDIVIR, VIRODIN 400 mg cap.
12. **Nelfinavir:** 750 mg TDS; NELFIN, NELVIR, NEIVEX 250 mg tab.
13. **Ritonavir:** 600 mg BD to be taken with meal; 100 mg with each dose to boost another protease inhibitor;
    RITOVIR, RITOMUNE, RITOMAX 100 mg cap/tab.

14. **Saquinavir:** 1200 mg TDS oral taken with or just after a meal or 1000 mg BD along with ritonavir 100 mg; SAQUIN 300 mg cap.
15. **Lopinavir:** 400 mg (taken with ritonavir 100 mg) BD with food.
    RITOMAX-L, V-LETRA: Lopinavir 133.3 mg + Ritonavir 33.3 mg cap.
16. **Darunavir:** 600 mg along with ritonavir 100 mg twice daily; DARUVIR 300 mg tab.
17. **Raltegravir:** 400 mg BD; ISENTRESS 400 mg tab.
18. **Dolutegravir:** 50 mg OD, 50 mg BD in those taking enzyme inducers; INSTGRA, NAIVEX 50 mg tab.
19. **Bictegravir:** 50 mg once daily;
    TAFFIC: Bictegravir 50 mg + Emtricitabine 200 mg + tenofovir alafenamide 25 mg tab; one tab daily.

Some Antiretroviral Combinations

1. **Tenofovir** 300 mg + **Emtricitabine** 200 mg tab: TENVIR–EM, TAVIN-EM, TENOF-EM tabs.
2. **Tenofovir** 300 mg + **Lamivudine** 300 mg + **Efavirenz** 600 mg: TRIODAY tab.
3. **Lamivudine** 150 mg + **Zidovudine** 300 mg tab (1 tab BD);
   COMBIVIR, CYTOCOM, DUOVIR, LAMUZID tab.
4. **Lamivudine** 150 mg + **Zidovudine** 300 mg + **Nevirapine** 200 mg tab (1 tab BD);
   DUOVIR-N, CYTOCOM-N, NEXIVIR-Z.
5. **Lamivudine** 150 mg + **Zidovudine** 300 mg 2 tab and **Efavirenz** 600 mg 1 tab kit;
   CYTOCOM-E kit.

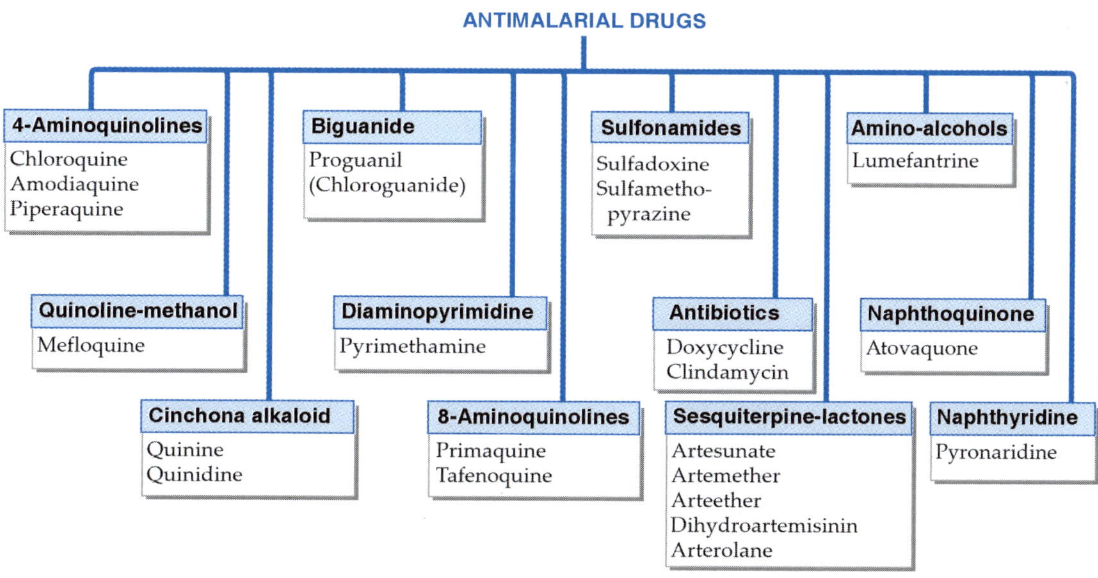
ANTIMALARIAL DRUGS
4-Aminoquinolines
Chloroquine
Amodiaquine
Piperaquine
Biguanide
Proguanil
(Chloroguanide)
Sulfonamides
Sulfadoxine
Sulfametho-
pyrazine
Amino-alcohols
Lumefantrine
Quinoline-methanol
Mefloquine
Diaminopyrimidine
Pyrimethamine
Antibiotics
Doxycycline
Clindamycin
Naphthoquinone
Atovaquone
Cinchona alkaloid
Quinine
Quinidine
8-Aminoquinolines
Primaquine
Tafenoquine
Sesquiterpine-lactones
Artesunate
Artemether
Arteether
Dihydroartemisinin
Arterolane
Naphthyridine
Pyronaridine

Preparations

1. **Chloroquine:** For clinical cure: 600 mg (base) followed by 300 mg after 8 hours and 300 mg daily for 2 days (total 1500 mg in 3 days) for infants 150 mg, children 1–4 years 200–400 mg, 5–10 years 600–1000 mg.

   For suppressive prophylaxis: 300 mg weekly (only in chloroquine sensitive *P. falciparum* areas).

   Chloroquine phosphate: (250 mg = 150 mg base): RESOCHIN 150 mg (base) tab; CLOQUIN, LARIAGO, NIVAQUIN-P 250 mg tab, 500 mg forte tab, 100 mg (base) per 10 ml oral susp.
2. **Amodiaquine:** For treatment of acute attack of malaria: 25–35 mg/kg over 3 days (used only as ACT combination therapy).
3. **Piperaquine:** 960 mg (16 mg/kg) along with dihydroartemisinin 120 mg (2 mg/kg) daily × 3 days (as ACT combination therapy).
4. **Mefloquine:** For treatment of uncomplicated falciparum malaria: 25 mg/kg split into 2 doses taken on 2 days along with 3 days artesunate (4 mg/kg/day) combination therapy (ACT); For prophylaxis: 5 mg/kg (max 250 mg) per week started 2 weeks before entering endemic area;

   MEFQUE, CONFAL, FACITAL 250 mg tab to be taken after meals with plenty of water.
5. **Quinine:** For complicated (Cerebral) malaria: 20 mg/kg diluted in 5% glucose and infused i.v. over 4 hours, followed by 10 mg/kg over 8 hours repeated every 8 hours till patient improves (regains consciousness), followed by oral therapy to complete 7 day course. For uncomplicated falciparum malaria: 600 mg (10 mg/kg) TDS oral for 7 days along with doxycycline 100 mg daily for 7 days or clindamycin 600 mg BD for 7 days;

   QUININE 300, 600 mg tab, 600 mg/2 ml inj; QUININGA 100 mg, 300 mg tabs, 300 mg/2 ml inj.
6. **Proguanil (chloroguanide):** For malaria prophylaxis: 200 mg daily with chloroquine 300 mg weekly till 4 weeks after exposure; PROGUNAL, LAVERAN 100 mg tab.

7. **Pyrimethamine-sulfadoxine:** For treatment of uncomplicated falciparum malaria: 75 mg + 1500 mg single dose as Sulfadoxine 500 mg + pyrimethamine 25 mg tab: LARIDOX, RIMODAR, FANCIDAR, MALOCIDE; REZIZ 500 mg + 25 mg tab and per 10 ml susp (adults 3 tab, children 9–14 yr 2 tab, 4–8 yr 1 tab, 1–4 yr ½ tab); REZIZ FORTE 750 mg + 37.5 mg tab.

   Sulfamethopyrazine 500 mg + **pyrimethamine** 25 mg tab: MALARWIN tab.
8. **Doxycycline:** For treatment of chloroquine resistant falciparum malaria: 100 mg OD combined with quinine.

   For prophylaxis of chloroquine resistant falciparum malaria in travellers: 100 mg OD (as alternative to mefloquine).
9. **Clindamycin:** 600 mg BD in combination with quinine for chloroquine resistant vivax/falciparum malaria.
10. **Primaquine:** For radical cure of vivax malaria: 15 mg (children 0.25 mg/kg) daily for 2 weeks along with chloroquine for 3 days; As gametocidal for falciparum malaria 45 mg (0.75 mg/kg) single dose along with chloroquine or ACT. MALIRID, LEOPRIME, EVAQUIN (as phosphate 26 mg = 15 mg base) 2.5, 7.5, 15, 45 mg tab.
11. **Artesunate:** oral (for uncomplicated falciparum malaria) 100 mg BD (4 mg/kg/day) × 3 days in combination with mefloquine or sulfadoxine-pyrimethamine as ACT.

    Parenteral (for severe and complicated falciparum malaria) 2.4 mg/kg i.v. or i.m. repeated after 12 and 24 hours and then once daily for 7 days. Switchover to oral ACT in-between whenever patient can take oral medication. FALCIGO, FALCYNATE 50 mg tab, 60 mg/vial inj., LARINATE, ARNATE 60 mg/vial inj.
12. **Artemether:** Oral (for uncomplicated falciparum malaria) 80 mg twice daily × 3 days in combination with lumefantrine as ACT (to be taken with fatty meal).

    Parenteral (for severe and complicated falciparum malaria) 3.2 mg/kg i.m. on 1st day, followed by 1.6 mg/kg daily for 7 days. Switch-over to 3 day oral ACT in-between whenever patient can take oral medication; PALUTHER, LARITHER, MALITHER 40 mg cap, 80 mg inj (in 1 ml arachis oil).
13. **Arteether:** (for severe and complicated falciparum malaria) 150 mg i.m. daily for 3 days (only for adults); Switch-over to 3 day oral ACT in-between whenever the patient is able to take oral medication. E-MAL, FALCY, RAPITHER-AB 150 mg/2 ml amp.

Artemisinin-based combination therapies (ACTs)

1. **Artemether-lumefantrine (1:6) (A/L):** Artemether (80 mg BD) + lumefantrine (480 mg BD) × 3 days
   COARTRIN, COMBITHER, LUMETHER (artemether 20 mg + lumefantrine 120 mg tab.) to be taken with fatty meal.
   Adult and child >35 kg 4 tab BD; child 25–35 kg 3 tab BD; 15–25 kg 2 tab BD; 5–15 kg 1 tab BD, all for 3 days.
   FALCIMAX PLUS, ARTE PLUS (artemether 80 mg + lumefantrine 480 mg tab) 1 tab BD × 3 days for adults.
2. **Artesunate-mefloquine (AS/MQ):** Artesunate 100 mg BD (4 mg / kg/day) × 3 days + mefloquine 750 mg (15 mg / kg) on 2nd day and 500 mg (10 mg / kg) on 3rd day (total 25 mg / kg).
   MEFLIAM PLUS: Artesunate 100 mg + mefloquine 200 mg pack of 6 FDC tabs; LARINATE-MF Kit: Artesunate 200 mg (3 tabs) + mefloquine 250 mg (6 tabs) kit; FALCIGO PLUS kit (Artesunate 100 mg tab + Mefloquine 200 mg tab kit)
3. **Artesunate-amodiaquine (AS/AQ):** Artesunate 200 mg (4 mg / kg) + amodiaquine 600 mg (10 mg / kg) per day × 3 days
   Artesunate 25 mg/50 mg/100 mg +Amodiaquine 67.5 mg/135 mg/270 mg fixed dose combination tablets;
   ASAQ 25 + 67.5 mg, 50 + 135 mg, 100 + 270 mg FDC tabs.
4. **Artesunate-sulfadoxine + pyrimethamine (AS-S/P):** Artesunate 100 mg BD (4 mg / kg/day) × 3 days + sulfadoxine 1500 mg (25 mg / kg) and pyrimethamine 75 mg (1.25 mg / kg) single dose.
   ZESUNATE kit, MASUNATE kit, FALCIART kit (Artesunate 100 mg × 6 tab + sulfadoxine 500 mg/pyrimethamine 25 mg × 3 tab kit)
5. **Dihydroartemisinin-piperaquine (DHA/PPQ 1:8):** DHA 120 mg (2 mg / kg) + piperaquine 960 mg (16 mg / kg) daily × 3 days; for children < 25 kg body weight, DHA not less than 2.5 mg / kg + piperaquine 20 mg / kg daily × 3 days.

FaL-DP: Dihydroartemisinin 40 mg + piperaquine 320 mg cap.; DYSURE: DHA 80 mg + piperaquine 640 mg per 5 ml suspension, and DHA 40 mg + PPQ 320 mg tab.

6. **Arterolane-piperaquine:** Arterolane (as maleate) 150 mg + piperaquine 750 mg daily × 3 days (approved only for adults).
SYNRIAM (arterolane 150 mg + piperaquine 750 mg) cap, 1 cap OD × 3 days

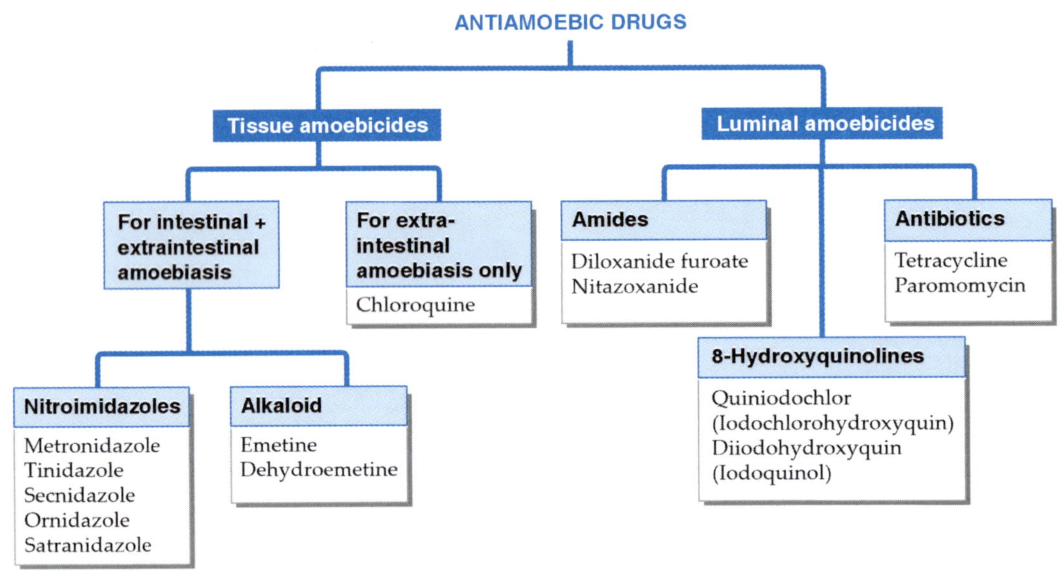
ANTIAMOEBIC DRUGS
Tissue amoebicides
Luminal amoebicides
For intestinal + extraintestinal amoebiasis
For extra-intestinal amoebiasis only
Chloroquine
Amides
Diloxanide furoate
Nitazoxanide
Antibiotics
Tetracycline
Paromomycin
8-Hydroxyquinolines
Quiniodochlor
(Iodochlorohydroxyquin)
Diiodohydroxyquin
(Iodoquinol)
Nitroimidazoles
Metronidazole
Tinidazole
Secnidazole
Ornidazole
Satranidazole
Alkaloid
Emetine
Dehydroemetine

Preparations

1. **Metronidazole:** *For amoebic dysentery and liver abscess*—800 mg TDS (children 30–50 mg/kg/day) for 7–10 days oral, or 500 mg slow i.v. infusion every 6–8 hours till oral therapy is instituted; *For mild intestinal amoebiasis*—400 mg TDS for 5–7 days. *For serious anaerobic bacterial infections*: 15 mg/kg infused i.v. over 1 hr followed by 7.5 mg/kg every 6 hrs till oral therapy can be instituted with 400–800 mg TDS;
   FLAGYL, METROGYL, METRON, ARISTOGYL 200, 400 mg tab, 200 mg/5 ml susp. (as benzoyl metronidazole: tasteless); 500 mg/100 ml i.v. infusion; UNIMEZOL 200, 400 mg tabs, METROGYL GEL, LUPIGYL GEL: 1% gel for vaginal/topical application.
2. **Tinidazole:** For *intestinal amoebiasis*: 2 g OD for 3 days (children 30–50 mg/kg/day) or 0.6 g BD for 5–10 days.
   Trichomoniasis and giardiasis: 2 g single dose or 0.6 g OD for 7 days.
   For *Anaerobic infections*:
   prophylactic—2 g single dose before colorectal surgery;
   therapeutic—2 g followed by 0.5 g BD for 5 days oral, 0.8 g i.v. infusion 8–12 hourly.
   For *H. pylori:* 500 mg BD for 1–2 weeks in triple combination;
   TINIBA 300, 500 mg tabs; 800 mg/400 ml i.v. infusion; FASIGYN 0.5 g and 1 g tab, TINI 0.3 g, 0.5 g tabs, 75 mg/5 ml and 150 mg/5 ml oral susp., TINVISTA 500 mg tab, AMEBAMAGMA 0.3 g and 0.5 g tabs.
3. **Secnidazole:** 2 g single dose (children 30 mg/kg) for intestinal amoebiasis, giardiasis, trichomonas vaginitis and nonspecific bacterial vaginosis; 1.5 g/day for 5 days in acute amoebic dysentery;
   SECNIL, SECZOL 0.5, 1.0 g tabs.
4. **Ornidazole:** 2 g OD oral for 3 days or 0.6 g BD for 5–10 days; 0.5–1.0 g slow i.v. infusion;
   DAZOLIC 500 mg tab, 500 mg/100 ml vial for i.v. infusion. ORNIDA 500 mg tab, 125 mg/5 ml susp.
5. **Satranidazole:** Amoebiasis: 300 mg BD for 3–5 days, giardiasis and trichomoniasis: 600 mg single dose orally;
   SATROGYL 300 mg tab.

6. **Emetine:** 60 mg i.m./s.c. OD for not more than 10 days.
7. **Dehydroemetine:** 60–100 mg i.m./s.c. OD for not more than 10 days;
   DEHYDROEMETINE HCL, TILEMETIN 30 mg/ml inj 1 and 2 ml amps.
8. **Chloroquine:** 600 mg (base) daily for 2 days followed by 300 mg OD for 2–3 weeks.
9. **Diloxanide furoate:** 500 mg TDS for 5–10 days; children 20 mg/kg/day;
   FURAMIDE, AMICLINE 0.5 g tab; in TINIBA–DF 250 mg + 150 mg tinidazole and TINIBA-DF FORTE 500 mg + 300 mg tabs.
10. **Nitazoxanide:** 500 mg (children 7.5 mg/kg) BD × 3 days.
    NITACURE, NITARID 200, 500 mg tabs, 100 mg/5 ml dry syrup.
11. **Quiniodochlor (Iodochlorohydroxyquin, Clioquinol):** 250–500 mg TDS;
    ENTEROQUINOL, QUINOFORM 250 mg tab.
12. **Tetracycline/Oxytetracycline:** 250 mg QID oral.

Drugs for Giardiasis

1. **Metronidazole:** 400 mg TDS (children 15 mg/kg/day) for 5–7 days or 2 g daily for 3 days.
2. **Tinidazole/Secnidazole:** 2 g single dose or 0.6 g daily for 7 days.
3. **Nitazoxanide:** 500 mg (children 7.5 mg/kg) BD × 3 days.
4. **Quiniodochlor:** 250 mg TDS for 7 days.
5. **Furazolidone:** 100 mg TDS for 5–7 days; FUROXONE 25 mg/5 ml susp.

Drugs for Trichomoniasis

A. Drugs used orally

1. **Metronidazole:** 400 mg TDS for 7 days or 2 g single dose.
2. **Tinidazole:** 600 mg OD for 7 days or 2 g single dose.
3. **Secnidazole:** 2 g single dose.

B. Drugs used intravaginally

1. **Quiniodochlor:** 200 mg inserted in the vagina every night for 1–3 weeks; GYNOSAN 200 mg vaginal tab.
2. **Metronidazole:** 2% topical gel applied in vagina once or twice daily; METROGYL GEL, LUPIGYL GEL 2% gel.
3. **Povidone-iodine:** 200 mg inserted in the vagina daily at night for 2 weeks; BETADINE VAGINAL 200 mg pessaries.

Drugs for Leishmaniasis (Kala azar)

1. **Amphotericin B deoxycholate:** 0.75–1.0 mg/kg i.v. infusion over 4 hours daily or on alternate days till 15 mg/kg total dose.
2. **Liposomal amphotericin B:** 10 mg/kg single dose i.v. infusion, or 3–5 mg/kg i.v. infusion daily for 3–5 days (total dose 15 mg/kg).
3. **Miltefosine:** Adults weighing >25 kg—50 mg cap twice daily orally; for adults weighing <25 kg—50 mg cap once daily; for children (2–11 years, body weight <25 kg) 2.5 mg/kg/day (as 10 mg caps). All doses given with meals for 28 days.
4. **Paromomycin sulfate:** 15 mg/kg i.m. OD for 21 days.
5. **Sodium stibogluconate:** 20 mg/kg i.m. or slow i.v. injection daily for 30 days (in areas with *Leishmania* sensitive to stibogluconate).

Combinations (Coadministered drugs)

1. Liposomal amphotericin B (5 mg/kg i.v. infusion single dose) + Miltefosine (oral as above for 7 days)
2. Liposomal amphotericin B (5 mg/kg i.v. infusion single dose) + Paromomycin (15 mg/kg i.m. daily for 10 days)
3. Miltefosine (oral as above for 10 days) + Paromomycin (15 mg/kg i.m. daily for 10 days).

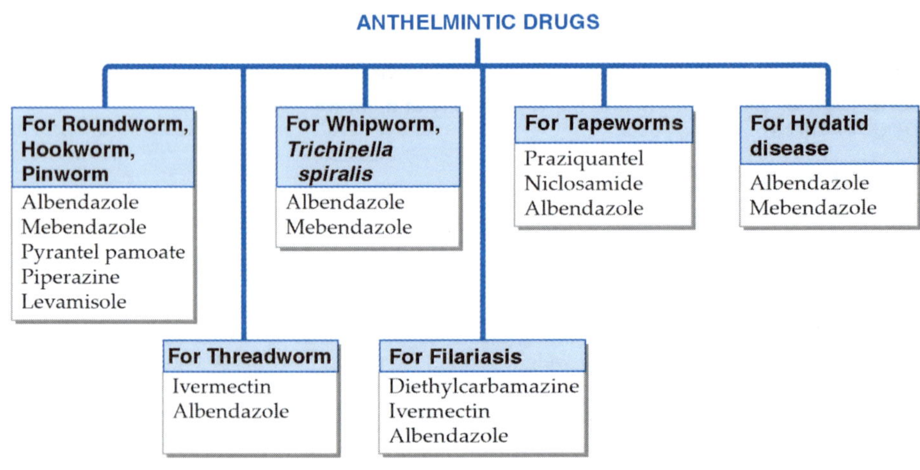

Preparations

1. **Mebendazole:** For round worm, hookworm and whipworm (*Trichuris)* 100 mg BD for 3 days; for pinworm 100 mg single dose repeated after 2–3 weeks; for *Trichinella spiralis* 200 mg BD for 4 days; for hydatid disease 200–400 mg BD–TDS for 3–4 weeks; children 1–2 year age 1/2 dose;
   MEBEX, WORMIN 100 mg chewale tab, 100 mg/5 ml susp, MEBAZOLE 100 mg tab.
2. **Albendazole:** For roundworm, hookworm, pinworm and whipworm 400 mg single dose (for children 1–2 years 1/2 dose); for tapeworms, strongyloidosis and trichinosis 400 mg daily for 3 days; neurocysticercosis 15 mg/kg daily for 8–15 days (along with corticosteroids); hydatid disease 400 mg BD for 4 weeks (upto 3 courses with 2 weeks gap); ZENTEL, COMBANTRIN-A, ALMINTH, ALBEZOLE 400 mg tab, 200 mg/5 ml susp.
3. **Pyrantel pamoate:** For roundworm, *Ancylostoma* and pinworm 10 mg/kg single dose, for *Necator* and strongyloidosis 10 mg/kg daily for 3 days; NEMOCID, PYMOLAR, EXPENT 250 mg tab, 500 mg/10 ml susp.
4. **Piperazine:** For roundworm infestation 4 g once a day for 2 consecutive days; children 0.75 g/year of age (max. 4 g). Enterobiasis—50 mg/kg (max. 2 g) once a day for 7 days or 75 mg/kg (max. 4 g) single dose, repeated after 3 weeks.
   PIPERAZINE CITRATE; 0.75 g/5 ml elixir in 30 ml, 115 ml bottle; 0.5 g (as phosphate) tablets.
5. **Levamisole:** For roundworm 150 mg (adults), 100 mg (children 20–39 kg body weight), 50 mg (children 10–19 kg weight) single dose, for *Ancylostoma* 2 doses 12 hour apart;
   DEWORMIS, VERMISOL 50, 150 mg tabs, 50 mg/5 ml syr.
6. **Diethylcarbamazine citrate:** For filariasis 2 mg/kg TDS for 12–21 days, for tropical eosinophilia 2–4 mg/kg TDS for 2–3 weeks; HETRAZAN, BANOCIDE 50, 100 mg tabs, 120 mg/5 ml syr, 50 mg/5 ml pediatric syr.
7. **Ivermectin:** 10–15 mg (0.2 mg/kg) orally single dose for strongyloidosis, enterobiasis, ascariasis as well as for scabies and pediculosis; for filariasis and onchocerciasis 0.2 mg/kg is repeated annually along with albendazole 400 mg; IVERMECTOL, IVERMECT, VERMIN 3 mg, 6 mg tabs, to be taken on empty stomach.

8. **Niclosamide:** For tapeworm (*T. solium, T. saginata*) 2.0 g taken in 2 doses 1 hour apart (children 2–6 years 1.0 g total dose) followed by a saline purge after 2 hours; for *H. nana* 2.0 g repeated daily for 5 days; NICLOSAN 0.5 g tab (to be chewed and swallowed with water).
9. **Praziquantel:** For tapeworm (*T. solium, T. saginata*) 10 mg/kg single dose in the morning; for *H. nana* and *D. latum* 15–25 mg/kg single dose in the morning; for neurocysticercosis 50 mg/kg/day in 3 divided doses for 15 days; for Schistosomiasis 40–75 mg/kg in one day; for other flukes 75 mg/kg in one day for 1–2 days; CYSTICIDE 500 mg tab, DISTOCIDE 600 mg tab.

13 Anticancer Drugs (Antineoplastic Drugs)

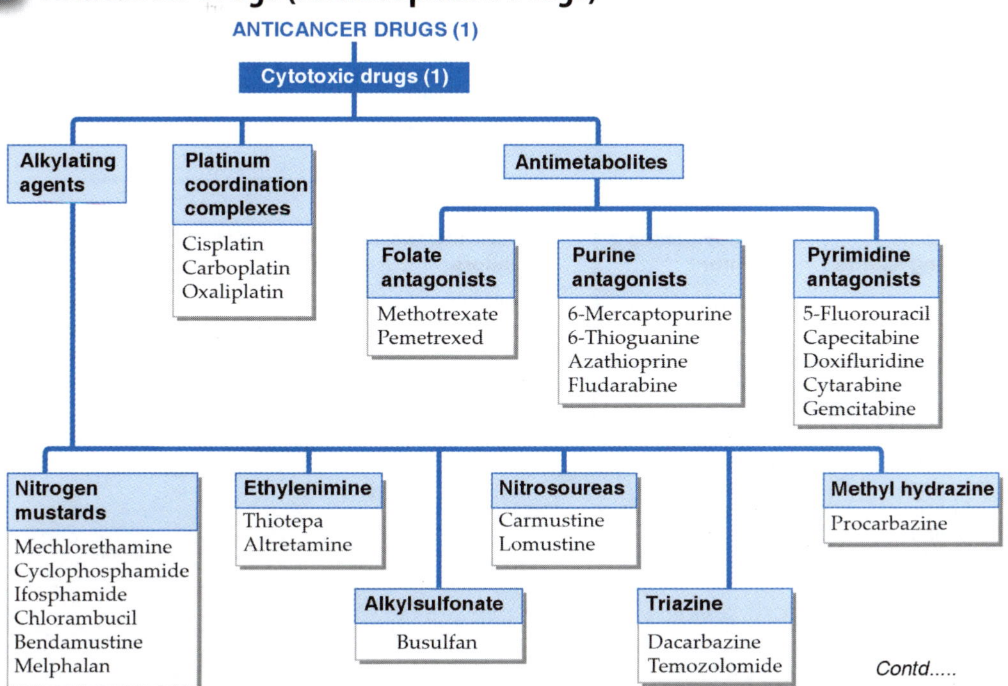

Contd.....

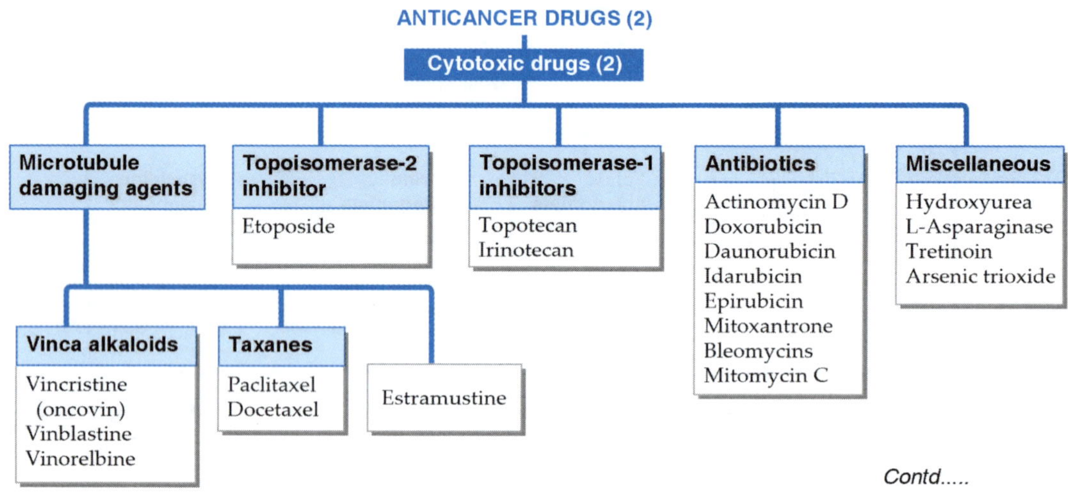
ANTICANCER DRUGS (2)
Cytotoxic drugs (2)
Microtubule damaging agents
Topoisomerase-2 inhibitor
Etoposide
Topoisomerase-1 inhibitors
Topotecan
Irinotecan
Antibiotics
Actinomycin D
Doxorubicin
Daunorubicin
Idarubicin
Epirubicin
Mitoxantrone
Bleomycins
Mitomycin C
Miscellaneous
Hydroxyurea
L-Asparaginase
Tretinoin
Arsenic trioxide
Vinca alkaloids
Vincristine (oncovin)
Vinblastine
Vinorelbine
Taxanes
Paclitaxel
Docetaxel
Estramustine

Contd.....

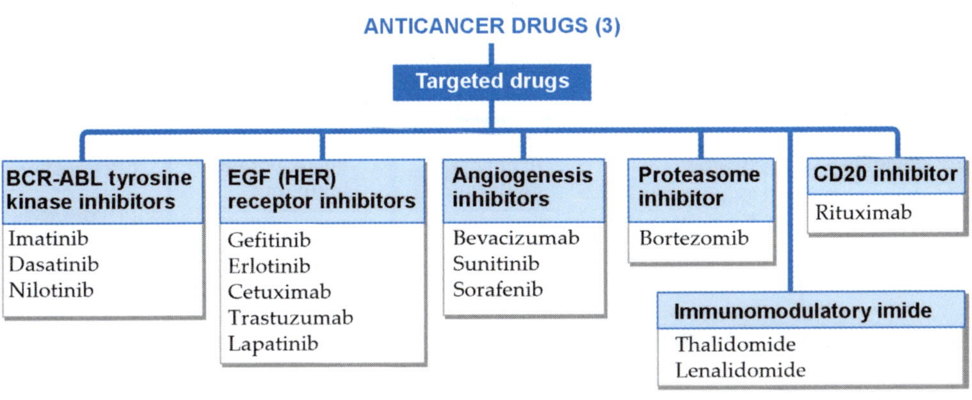

Contd.....

EGF: Epidermal growth factor

HER: Human epidermal growth factor receptor

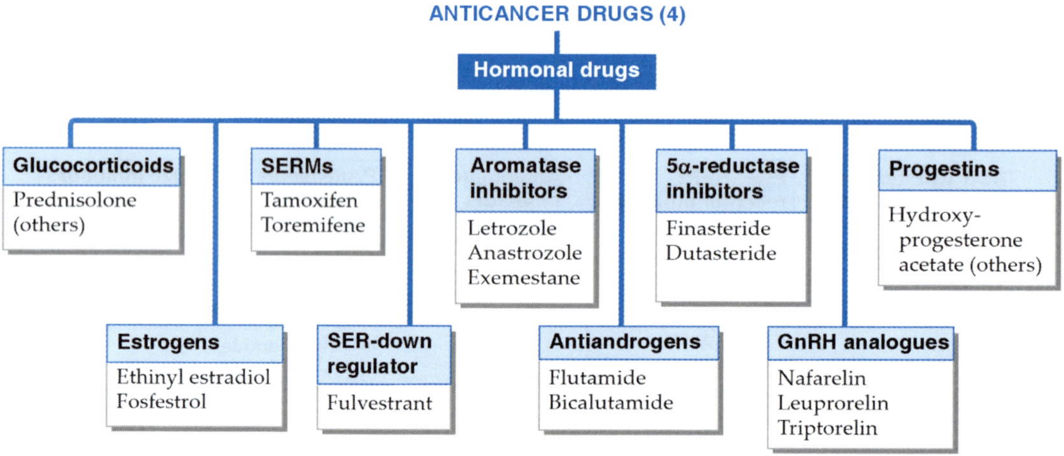

ANTICANCER DRUGS (4)

Hormonal drugs

- **Glucocorticoids**: Prednisolone (others)
- **Estrogens**: Ethinyl estradiol, Fosfestrol
- **SERMs**: Tamoxifen, Toremifene
- **SER-down regulator**: Fulvestrant
- **Aromatase inhibitors**: Letrozole, Anastrozole, Exemestane
- **Antiandrogens**: Flutamide, Bicalutamide
- **5α-reductase inhibitors**: Finasteride, Dutasteride
- **GnRH analogues**: Nafarelin, Leuprorelin, Triptorelin
- **Progestins**: Hydroxy-progesterone acetate (others)

SERMs: Selective estrogen receptor modulators

SER: Selective estrogen receptor

GnRH: Gonadotropin releasing hormone

Preparations

1. **Cyclophosphamide:** 2–3 mg/kg/day oral; 10–15 mg/kg i.v. every 7–10 days, i.m. use also possible; ENDOXAN, CYCLOXAN 50 mg tab; 200, 500, 1000 mg inj.
2. **Ifosfamide:** 10–15 mg/kg i.v.; IPAMIDE 1 g vial, HOLOXAN-UROMITEXAN 1 g vial + 3 amps of mesna 200 mg inj.
3. **Chlorambucil:** 4–10 mg (0.1–0.2 mg/kg) oral daily for 3–6 weeks, then 2 mg daily for maintenance; LEUKERAN 2, 5 mg tab.
4. **Melphalan:** 10 mg daily for 7 days or 6 mg/day for 2–3 weeks—4 weeks gap—2 to 4 mg daily for maintenance orally. Also used for regional perfusion in malignant melanoma; ALKERAN 2, 5 mg tab, 50 mg per vial for inj.
5. **Bendamustine:** 100–120 mg/m^2 i.v. daily for 2 days in 28 days cycles; XYOTIN 100 mg/vial inj.
6. **Altretamine:** 260 mg/m^2/day oral in 4 divided doses for 2–3 weeks; CANTRET 50 mg cap.
7. **Busulfan:** 2–6 mg/day (0.06 mg/kg/day) orally; MYLERAN, BUSUPHAN 2 mg tab.
8. **Lomustine (CCNU):** 100–130 mg/m^2 BSA single oral dose every 6 weeks; LOMUSTINE, MOOSTIN 40, 100 mg cap.
9. **Dacarbazine (DTIC):** For malignant melanoma 3.5 mg/kg/day i.v. for 10 days, repeat after 4 weeks; for Hodgkin's disease 3.5 mg/kg i.v. on day 1 and 15 of 4 weeks cycles; DACARIN 100, 200, 500 mg inj; DACARZINE 200 mg/vial inj.
10. **Temozolamide:** 100–250 mg/day; GLIOZ, GLIOGREY 20, 100, 250 mg caps, 100 mg/vial inj.
11. **Procarbazine:** 100 mg/$m^{2/}$day for 14 days in 28 day cycles; INDICARB 20 mg cap, NEOZINE, P-CARZINE 50 mg cap.
12. **Cisplatin:** 50–100 mg/m^2 BSA by slow i.v. infusion every 3–4 weeks; CISPLATIN, CISPLAT, PLATINEX 10 mg/10 ml, 50 mg/50 ml vial.
13. **Carboplatin:** 400 mg/m^2 as i.v. infusion over 15–60 min, to be repeated only after 4 weeks; ONCOCARBIN, KEMOCARB 150 mg, 450 mg/vial inj.

14. **Oxaliplatin:** 85 mg/m^2 i.v. every 2 weeks; KINAPLAT, OPLATIN 50 mg in 25 ml and 100 mg in 50 ml vial.
15. **Methotrexate:** 15–30 mg/day for 5 days orally or 20–40 mg/m^2 body surface area (BSA) i.m./i.v. twice weekly, maintenance therapy 2.5–15 mg/day;
NEOTREXATE 2.5 mg tab, 50 mg/2 ml inj; BIOTREXATE 2.5 mg tab, 5, 15, 50 mg/vial inj, FOLITREX 2.5 mg, 5 mg, 7.5 mg, 10 mg, 15 mg tabs; 15 mg/ml and 50 mg/2 ml inj.
16. **Pemetrexed:** 500 mg/m^2 i.v. every 3 weeks;
PEMEX 500 mg vial for i.v. inj, PEXITAZ 100 mg, 500 mg per vial inj.
17. **6-Mercaptopurine:** 2.5 mg/kg/day orally, half dose for maintenance;
PURINETHOL, EMPURINE, 6-MP, MERCAPTO 50 mg tab.
18. **6-Thioguanine:** 100–200 mg/m^2/day oral for 5–20 days; 6–TG 40 mg tab.
19. **Azathioprine:** 3–5 mg/kg/day oral, maintenance 1–2 mg/kg/day;
IMURAN, AZOPRINE, AZORAN 50 mg tab.
20. **Fludarabine:** 25 mg/m^2 BSA daily for 5 days every 28 days by i.v. infusion, FLUDARA 50 mg/vial inj.
21. **Fluorouracil (5-FU):** 500 mg/m^2 i.v. infusion over 1–3 hours weekly for 6–8 weeks, or 12 mg/kg/day i.v. for 4 days followed by 6 mg/kg i.v. on alternate days 3–4 doses;
FLURACIL, FIVOCIL 250 mg/5 ml and 500 mg/10 ml vial for i.v. inj.
22. **Capecitabine:** 2.5 g/m^2 in 2 divided doses daily with meals for 2 weeks, repeat after one week gap;
CAPIIBINE, CAPXCEL 150 mg, 500 mg tabs.
23. **Doxifluridine:** 800 mg TDS: CORCIDOX 200 mg cap.
24. **Cytarabine:** 100 mg/m^2 i.v. injection 2–3 times/day for 5–10 days, or 1–3 g/day i.v.
REMCYTA, CYTROSAR, CYTABIN, BIOBIN 100, 500, 1000 mg inj.
25. **Gemcitabine:** 1 g/m^2 i.v. infusion (10 mg/min) every week for upto 7 weeks;
CELGEM, GEMTAZ, ONCOGEM 200 mg and 1000 mg/vial inj.

26. Vincristine (Oncovin): 1.5–2 mg/m^2 BSA i.v. weekly; ONCOCRISTIN, CYTOCRISTIN 1 mg/vial inj.
27. Vinblastine: 0.1–0.15 mg/kg i.v. weekly × 3 doses; UNIBLASTIN, CYTOBLASTIN 10 mg/vial inj.
28. Vinorelbine: 25–30 mg/m^2 weekly by slow i.v. inj over 10 min; VINOTEC, RELBOVIN, ONCOBINE 10 mg, 50 mg/vial inj.
29. Paclitaxel: 135–175 mg/m^2 by i.v. infusion over 3 hr, repeated every 3 weeks; ALTAXEL, MITOTAX, ONCOTAXEL 30, 100, 260 mg as 6 mg/ml in cremophor (polyoxyethylated castor oil + alcohol + water) emulsion.
30. Docetaxel: 75–100 mg/m^2 i.v. over 1 hr; repeat at 3 weeks; DOCECAD, DOCETERE, DOXEL 20, 80, 120 mg/vial inj.
31. Estramustine: 4–5 mg/kg oral TDS; ESMUST, ESTRAM 140 mg cap.
32. Etoposide: 50–100 mg/m^2/day i.v. for 5 days, 100–200 mg/day oral; PELTASOL 100 mg in 5 ml inj., LASTET 25, 50, 100 mg cap, 100 mg/5 ml inj, ACTITOP 50, 100 mg caps, 100 mg/5 ml inj.
33. Topotecan: 1.5 mg/m^2 i.v. over 30 min daily for 5 days in 3 week or 4 week cycles; TOPOTEC, CANTOP 2.5 mg inj.
34. Irinotecan: 125 mg/m^2 i.v. over 90 min weekly for 4 weeks in 6 weeks cycles. IRINOTEL, IRNOCAM 40 mg (2 ml), 100 mg (5 ml) inj.
35. Actinomycin D (Dactinomycin): 15 μg/kg i.v. daily for 5 days; DACMOZEN 0.5 mg/vial inj.
36. Daunorubicin (Rubidomycin): 25–50 mg/m^2 BSA i.v. daily for 3 days, repeat after 3–4 weeks. DAUNOCIN, DAUNOMYCIN 20 mg/vial inj.
37. Doxorubicin: 60–75 mg/m^2 BSA slow i.v. injection every 3 weeks; ADRIAMYCIN, DOXORUBICIN, ONCODRIA 10 mg, 50 mg per vial inj.
38. Epirubicin: 60–90 mg/m^2 i.v. over 5 min, repeated at 3 weeks; total dose <900 mg/m^2. ALRUBICIN, EPIRUBITEC 10, 50 mg vials for reconstitution with diluent provided.

39. **Idarubicin:** 12 $mg/m^2/day$ for 3 days by slow i.v. injection; ZAVEDOS 5 mg/vial, 10 mg/vial inj.
40. **Mitoxantrone:** 14 mg/m^2 single i.v. dose, repeat at 3 weeks; ONCOTRON 20 mg/10 ml inj.
41. **Bleomycin:** 30 mg twice weekly i.v. or i.m. (total dose not to exceed 250 mg); BLEOCIN, ONCOBLEO 15 mg inj.
42. **Mitomycin C:** 10 mg/m^2 BSA, infused i.v. in one day; MITOCIN, ALMITO 2, 10 mg inj.
43. **Hydroxyurea:** 20–30 mg/kg daily or 80 mg/kg twice weekly oral; CYTODROX, HONDREA, UNIDREA 500 mg cap.
44. **L-Asparaginase:** 50–200 KU/kg i.v. or i.m. twice weekly for 3–4 weeks; LEUNASE, HOILASP 10,000 KU per vial inj.
45. **Imatinib:** 400 mg/day with meals; for accelerated phase of CML 600-800 mg/day; IMATIB-α, SHANTINIB, GLIVEC 100 mg caps; UNITINIB 100, 400 mg caps.
46. **Dasatinib:** 100–400 mg/day; DISANAT 20 mg, 50 mg tabs, INVISTA 50 mg, 100 mg tabs.
47. **Nilotinib:** 150–200 mg/day; TASIGNA 150, 200 mg tab, TAKVEO 200 mg tab.
48 **Gefitinib:** 250 mg/day oral; GEFONIB, GEFTINAT 250 mg tab/cap.
49. **Erlotinib:** 100–150 mg OD 1 hour before or 2 hours after meal; ERLOTEC, ERLONAT 100, 150 mg tabs.
50. **Cetuximab:** 400 mg/m^2 slow i.v. infusion loading dose, followed by 250 mg/m^2 i.v. every week; ERBITUX 100 mg in 50 ml inj.
51. **Trastuzumab:** 2–8 mg/kg i.v. infusion once every week; HERCEPTIN 440 mg in 50 ml inj.
52. **Lapatinib:** 1250–1500 mg/day; TYKERB 250 mg tab.
53. **Bevacizumab:** 5–10 mg/kg i.v. infusion over 30–90 min. AVASTIN 100 mg, 400 mg per vial inj.

54. **Sunitinib:** 37.5–50 mg OD oral; SUTENT 12.5 mg, 25 mg, 50 mg caps.
55. **Sorafenib:** 400 mg twice daily; may be reduced to 400 mg once daily; SORANIB, NEXAVAR 200 mg tab.
56. **Bortezomib:** 1.3 mg/m^2 i.v. bolus injection, 4 doses at 3 day intervals;
    EGYBORT 3.5 mg/vial inj; MYEZOM 2 mg, 3.5 mg/vial inj.
57. **Rituximab:** Initially 50–375 mg/m^2 slow i.v. infusion, followed by 500 mg/m^2;
    REDITUX 100 mg, 500 mg per vial inj.
58. **Lenalidomide:** For multiple myeloma—25 mg OD for 21 days—7 day gap in 28 day cycles;
    For myelodysplastic syndromes—10 mg OD; modify dose according response.
    LENALID, LIDOMIDE, LYNIDE, LENANGIO 10 mg, 25 mg caps.

Note: *See* Index for preparations of hormones and hormone antagonists

14 Miscellaneous Drugs

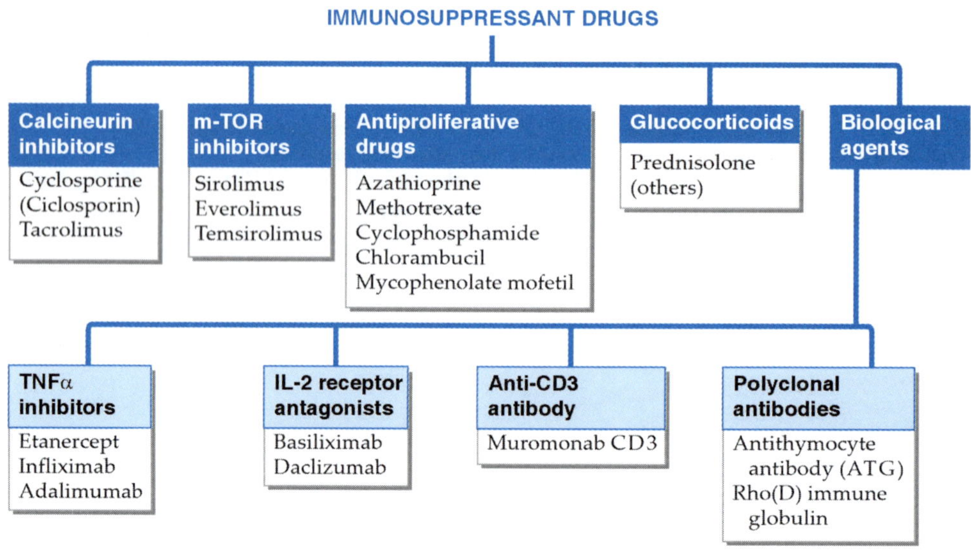

Preparations

1. **Cyclosporine:** 10–15 mg/kg/day with milk or fruit juice till 1–2 weeks after transplantation, gradually reduced to maintenance dose of 2–6 mg/kg/day. Therapy may be started with 3–5 mg/kg i.v. infusion. IMUSPORIN, GRAFTIN SOFGEL 25, 50, 100 mg soft gelatin cap; microemulsion formulation SANDIMMUN NEORAL, PANIMUN BIORAL 25, 50, 100 mg caps; SANDIMMUN, PANIMUN 100 mg/ml inj in 1 ml, 5 ml, 50 ml vials dispersed in cremaphor emulsion: to be diluted and infused i.v. over 4–6 hours.
2. **Tacrolimus:** 0.05–0.1 mg/kg 12 hourly oral (for renal transplantation) 0.1–0.2 mg/kg BD (for liver transplantation); PANGRAF, TACROMUS 0.5, 1.0, 5.0 mg caps; TACRODERM, TACREL 0.03, 0.1% oint.
3. **Sirolimus:** Loading dose 1 mg/m^2 orally daily, followed by titrated lower doses for maintenance; RAPACAN 1 mg tab.
4. **Everolimus:** 0.5–1 mg BD to prevent transplant rejection; 5–10 mg/day for treatment of certain malignancies; CERTICAN 0.25, 0.5, 0.75 mg tabs., AFINITOR, EVERTOR 5 mg, 10 mg tabs.
5. **Temsirolimus:** 25 mg i.v. once a week; TORISEL 25 mg/vial inj.
6. **Azathioprine:** Initially 3–5 mg/kg/day oral, followed by 1–2 mg/kg/day for maintenance.
7. **Cyclophosphamide:** 10–15 mg/kg i.v., 2–3 mg/kg/day oral.
8. **Methotrexate:** Initially 15–30 mg/day oral, 2.5–15 mg/day for maintenance.
9. **Chlorambucil:** 2–10 mg/day oral.
10. **Mycophenolate mofetil:** 1 g oral twice daily; CELLMUNE, MYCEPT, MYCOPHEN 250, 500 mg tab/cap.
11. **Infliximab:** 3–5 mg/kg infused i.v. every 4–8 weeks; REMICADE 100 mg/vial inj.

12. **Adalimumab:** 40 mg s.c. every 2 weeks; ADFRAR, EXEMPTIA, MABVINTRA 40 mg/0.8 ml inj.
13. **Etanercept:** 25–50 mg s.c. once or twice weekly; ENBREL, ENBROL 25 mg in 0.5 ml and 50 mg in 1 ml inj.
14. **Basiliximab:** 20 mg i.v. inj; SIMULECT 20 mg/vial inj.
15. **Antithymocyte globulin:** LYMPHOGLOBULIN (equine) 100 mg/vial inj.; 10 mg/kg/day i.v.; THYMOGLOBULIN (rabbit) 25 mg/vial inj.; 1.5 mg/kg/day; ATG 100 mg inj; 200 mg i.v./day.
16. **Rho(D) immune globulin:** 250–350 µg i.m. of freez dried preparation. RHESUMAN, RHOGAM 300 µg per vial and prefilled syringe.

Note: *See* Index for preparations of other drugs.

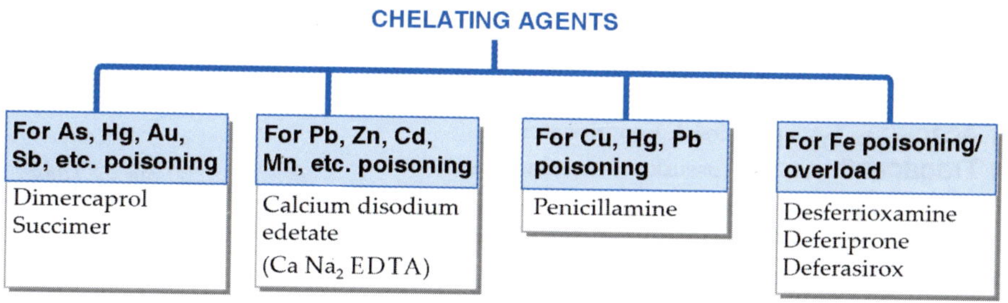

1. **Dimercaprol (British Antilewisite, BAL):** 5 mg/kg, followed by 2–3 mg/kg every 4–8 hours for 2 days, and then once daily for 10 days, injected i.m.; BAL INJ 100 mg/2 ml in arachis oil inj.
2. **Calcium disodium edetate (Ca Na_2 EDTA):** 1 g diluted in 200–300 ml saline and infused i.v. over 1 hour twice daily for 3–5 days, to be repeated after a week.
3. **Penicillamine:** 0.5–1 g daily in divided doses 1 hour before or 2 hour after meals to avoid chelation of dietary metals; ARTAMIN 150, 250 mg cap; PENICITIN, AARAMINE 250 mg cap.
4. **Desferrioxamine:** *For acute iron poisoning:* 0.5–1 g (50 mg/kg) i.m. 4–12 hourly as required or 10–15 mg/kg/hour (max 75 mg/kg in one day) i.v. infusion; *for transfusion siderosis in thalassemia patients* 0.5–1 g/day i.m.; DESFERAL 0.5 g/vial inj.
5. **Deferiprone:** 50–100 mg/kg oral daily in 2–4 divided doses; KELFER 250, 500 mg caps.
6. **Deferasirox:** *For chronic iron overload*—20 mg/kg OD on empty stomach; no food for next 1 hour. Dose to be adjusted later according to serum ferritin level.
   DESIROX, DEFRIJET 250 mg, 500 mg tabs; tablet to be dispersed in water/orange juice before taking.

LOCALLY ACTING DRUGS ON SKIN AND MUCOUS MEMBRANES

Demulcents

1. Gum Acacia: as 2–4% pseudosolution in water.
2. Gum Tragacanth: as 2–4% pseudosolution in water.
3. Glycyrrhiza: as glycyrrhiza dry extract 1–2 g or liquid extract 2–4 ml, in lozenges and mixtures.
4. Methylcellulose: 0.5% in nose drops and contact lens solution; CADILOSE 0.5% drops in 10 ml bottle.
5. Propylene glycol: 50% in water.
6. Glycerine: 10–50% in water.

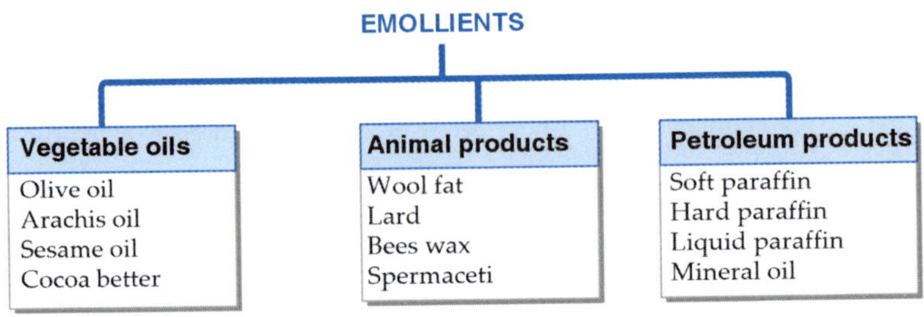

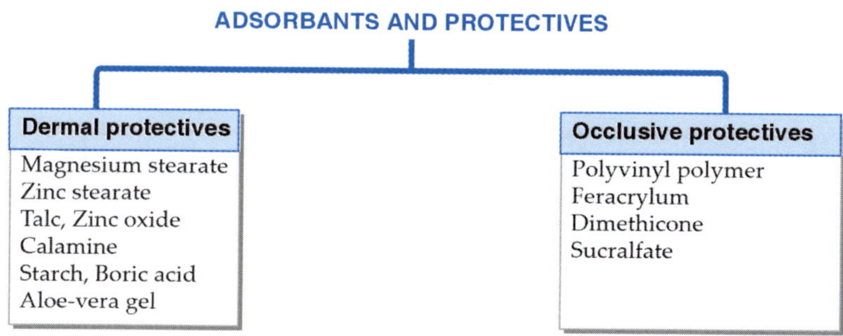

Preparations

CALADRYL: Calamine 8% diphenhydramine 1%, Camphor 0.1% lotion.
CALAK, CALMIS (Calamine lotion): Calamine 15%, zinc oxide 5%, bentonite 3%, sodium citrate 0.5%, liquified phenol 0.5%, glycerin 5% lotion.
CALACREME: Calamine 5% cream, CALAMINOL: Calamine 5% emulsion.
ALOVIT: Aloe extract 10%, Vit E 0.5% cream.
ALOEDERM: Aloe juice 10%, vit E acetate 0.2%, sesame oil 2% cream.
JULA: Aloe vera juice gel 50% gel.
LUBRIDERM-SF: Dimethicone 4%, vit E acetate 1%, vegetable oil 2%, propylene glycol 10% cream.
HEALEX SPRAY: Polyvinyl polymer 2.5% + benzocaine 0.36% as aerosol wound dressing.
SEPGARD GEL: Feracrylum 1% gel, to be applied as a thin film on the abrasion/wound.
SILENT-SF: White soft paraffin 2.5%, dimethicone 0.5% cream.
BARRIER-SF: Dimethicone 15%, vita E acetate 0.18% cream.
PEPSIGARD LIGHT GEL: Sucralfate 10% gel.

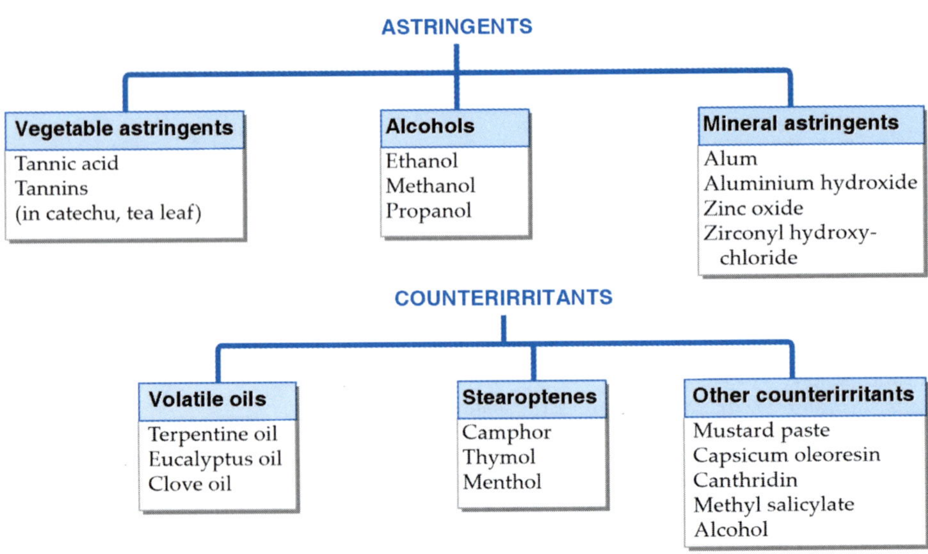
ASTRINGENTS
Vegetable astringents
Tannic acid
Tannins
(in catechu, tea leaf)
Alcohols
Ethanol
Methanol
Propanol
Mineral astringents
Alum
Aluminium hydroxide
Zinc oxide
Zirconyl hydroxy-chloride
COUNTERIRRITANTS
Volatile oils
Terpentine oil
Eucalyptus oil
Clove oil
Stearoptenes
Camphor
Thymol
Menthol
Other counterirritants
Mustard paste
Capsicum oleoresin
Canthridin
Methyl salicylate
Alcohol

Preparations

ALGIPAN: Capsicum oleoresin 0.1%, histamine 0.1%, methyl nicotinate 1%, glycol salicylate 5% cream.
RELISPRAY: Wintergreen oil (methyl salicylate) 20%, clove oil 1%, Menthol 4%, Nilgiri oil 6%, Camphor 10%, Cinnamon oil 0.5%, terpentine oil 10% spray
ARJET SPRAY: Methyl salicylate 875 mg, menthol 1.6 g, camphor 1.5 g, benzyl nicotinate 20 mg, squalance 250 mg, glycol salicylate 875 mg per 50 ml spray.
RELAXYL: Capsicum oleoresin 0.05%, mephenesin 10%, methyl nicotinate 1% ointment.
VICKS VAPORUB: Menthol 2.8%, camphor 5.25%, thymol 0.1% turpentine oil 5.5% ointment.
IODEX: Methylsalicylate 5%, iodine 4% nonstaining ointment.
AMRUTANJAN: Eucalyptus oil 17%, camphor 10%, thymol 1%, menthol 4.5%, methylsalicylate 7% ointment.
CAPSIGYL-D: Capsaicin 0.075%, methyl salicylate 20%, menthol 10%, camphor 5%, eucalyptus oil 5%, diclofenac 1% gel.

Keratolytics and Caustics

Salicylic acid,
Silver nitrate,
Glacial acetic acid
Resorcinol,
Phenol,
Podophyllum resin,
Trichloracetic acid,

Preparations

COSALIC: Salicylic acid 3%, coal tar 6% oint.
CLONVS-S: Sclicylic acid 3%, clobetasol 0.05% oint.
FOOT POWDER: Salicylic acid 2% dusting powder.
WHITFIELDS OINTMENT: Salicylic acid 3%, benzoic acid 6% oint.
PODOWART: Podophyllum resin 20% paint.
CONDYLINE: Podophyllotoxin 0.5% solution.
SALACTIN: Salicylic acid 16.7% + lactic acid 16.7% in flexible collodion paint; to be painted on the corn, avoiding normal skin.

Antiseborrheics

Selenium sulfide, Zinc pyrithione, Ketoconazole, Clotrimazole, Coal tar, Topical corticosteroids.

Preparations

SELSUN: Slenium sulfide 2.5% susp.
SELDRUFF PLUS: Selenium sulfide 2.5%, clotrimazole 1% susp.
SCALPE: Zinc pyrithione 1%, ketoconazole 2% shampoo.
KETOVATE, NIZRAL, OCONA: Ketoconazole 2% cream, 2% shampoo.
CANDID-TV SUSP: Selenium disulfide 2.5%, clotrimazole 1% susp.

Melanizing agents

1. Psoralen: 10–20 mg (0.3–0.6 mg/kg) orally followed 2 hours later by 15–30 min of exposure to sunlight/UV light; 0.25–1% local application on vitiliginous lesion followed by 1 min (initially) exposure to sunlight; exposure time is increased gradually as tolerated; MANADERM 10 mg tab, 1% oint.
2. Methoxsalen: MACSORALEN 10 mg tab, 1% solution, MELANOCYL 10 mg tab, 0.75% solution. Use similar to psoralen.
3. Trioxsalen: NEOSORALEN 5, 25 mg tabs, 0.2% lotion. Use similar to psoralen.

Demelanizing agents

1. Hydroquinone: 2–6% topical application; HYDE CREAM Hydroquinone 3% cream, MELALITE: Hydroquinone 2% with glycerylester of PABA 2.8% cream, ELOSONE–HT: Hydroquinone 2%, tretinoin 0.025%, mometasone 0.1% cream.
2. Monobenzone: 5–20% topical application; BENOQUIN 20% oint.
3. Azelaic acid: 10–20% topical application; AZIDERM 10%, 20% cream.

Sunscreens

1. *Chemical sunscreens*
   Para-aminobenzoic acid (PABA): 5–10% topical application; PABALAK 5% solution, PARAMINOL 10% cream.
   Oxybenzone: 2–6% topical application.
   Octyl methoxy cinnamate: 5% topical application;
   EUKROMA-SG: Oxybenzone 3%, Octyl methoxycinnamate 5%, hydroquinone 2% cream. SUNSTOP: octyl methoxycinnamate 7.5% + zinc oxide 7.5% gel.
   SUNSHIELD: Octyl methoxycinnamae 5% , Vit E 0.25% lotion.
2. *Physical sunscreens*
   Petroleum jelly (heavy), Titanium dioxide, Zinc oxide, Calamine
   MELASCREEN: Titanium dioxide, Zinc oxide, Octyl methoxy-cinnamate, benzophenone, avobenzone lotion/cream.

Drugs for Psoriasis

1. Topical corticosteroids: (*See* p. 47, 49)
2. Calcipotriol: 0.005% twice daily topical application on the lesions only; DAIVONEX 0.005% oint.
3. Tazarotene: 0.05-0.1% topical application daily in the evening; LATEZ 0.05%, 0.1% gel; TAZRET 0.05%, 0.1% cream.
4. Coaltar: 1–6% topical application;
   TARSYL: Coaltar 1%, Salicylic acid 3% lotion; COLAT-S coal tar 1%, salicylic acid 3% soap; SEBOTAR coal tar 2%, salicylic acid 0.5% soap.
5. Acitretin: 0.5–0.75 mg/kg/day oral; ACROTAC, ACTOID, ACERET 10, 25 mg tabs.
6. Psoralen-ultraviolet A (PUVA) therapy
7. *Immunosuppressants:* Methotrexate, Etanercept, Infliximab.
8. Apremilast: 10 mg BD initially, titrate to maintenance dose of 30 mg BD; APREZO, APRAIZO 10 mg, 20 mg, 30 mg tabs. PDLAST 30 mg tab.

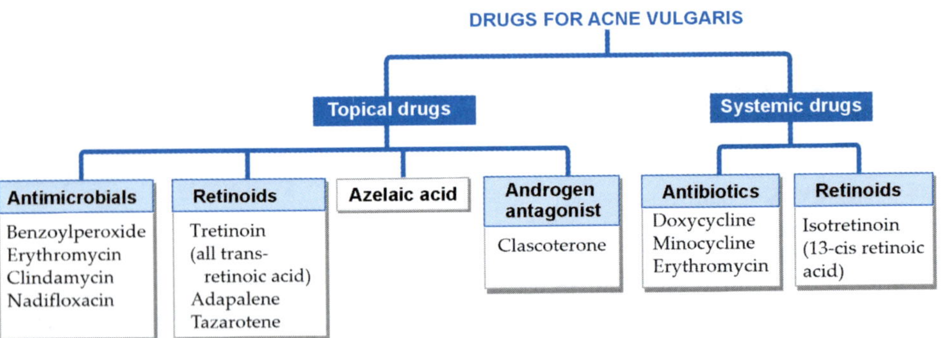

Preparations

1. Benzoyl peroxide: 2.5–10% topical application; PERSOL, PERNOX, BENZAC-AC 2.5% and 5% gel; in PERSOL FORTE 10% cream with sulfur ppt. 5%.
2. Tretinoin (Retinoic acid, all trans vitamin A acid): 0.025%–0.05% topical application; EUDYNA 0.05% cream, RETINO-A 0.025% and 0.05% cream.
3. Adapalene: 0.1% topical application once daily at bed time; ADAFERIN, ADAPEN, ACLENE 0.1% gel.
4. Azelaic acid: 10–20% topical application; AZIDERM 10%, 20% cream.
5. Erythromycin: 2–4% topical application; ACNEDERM 2% lotion and oint; ERYTOP 3% lotion and cream; ACNELAK-Z 4% lotion and gel with zinc acetate 2%, ACNESOL 2% lotion, 4% gel.

6. **Clindamycin:** 1% topical application; CLINDAC-A, CLINCIN, ACNESOL 1% gel.
7. **Nadifloxacin:** 1% topical application; NADIBACT, NADOXIN 1% topical cream.
8. **Clascoterone:** 1% topical application; WINLEVI 1% cream.
9. **Isotretinoin (13-cis retinoic acid)** 0.5–1 mg/kg/day; ISOTRETIN, SOTRET 10, 20 mg cap.

ANTISEPTICS AND DISINFECTANTS

1. *Phenol derivatives*:
   Phenol, Cresol, Hexylresorcinol, Chloroxylenol, Hexachlorophene.
2. *Oxidizing agents*:
   Pot. permangnate, Hydrogen peroxide, Benzoyl peroxide.
3. *Halogens*:
   Iodine, Iodophores (Povidone iodine), Chlorine, Chlorophores (Bleaching powder, Sod. hypochlorite).
4. *Biguanide*
   Chlorhexidine.
5. *Quaternary ammonium (Cationic);*
   Cetrimide, Benzalkonium chloride, Dequalinium chloride.
6. *Soaps*
   of Sod. and Pot.
7. *Alcohols*
   Ethanol, Isopropanol.
8. *Aldehydes*
   Formaldehyde, Glutaraldehyde.

9. *Acids*
   Boric acid
10. *Metallic salts*
    Silver nitrate, Silver sulfadiazine, Zinc sulfate, Calamine, Zinc oxide.
11. *Dyes*
    Gentian violet, Acriflavine, Proflavine.
12. *Furan derivative*
    Nitrofurazone.

Preparations

1. Phenol: 1–5%
2. Cresol: 0.5–4%; LYSOL 50% emulsion of cresol.
3. Chloroxylenol: 0.5–5%; DETTOL 4.8% solution, 0.8% cream, 0.8% soap, 1.4% lubricating obstetric cream, DETTOLIN 1% mouthwash
4. Hexachlorophene: 0.2–3.0% in soaps, dusting powder, etc.
5. Potassium permangnate: as 1:4000–1:10,000 aqueous solution (Condy's lotion).
6. Hydrogen peroxide: 3–10%
7. Iodine: 2% as Tincture iodine (alcoholic solution), 1.25% in Mandel's throat paint; IODEX 4% nonstaining oint.
8. Povidone iodine: 1–10%;
   BETADINE 5% solution, 5% ointment, 5% cream, 7.5% scrub solution, 5% powder, 200 mg vaginal pessary; PIODIN 10% solution, 10% cream, 1% mouth wash.

9. **Chlorine:** 0.2–0.4 parts per million (ppm).
10. **Chlorinated lime:** BLEACHING POWDER (30% chlorine).
11. **Sodium hypochlorite:** 4–6% solution.
12. **Chlorhexidine:** 0.1–1.5% solution; CHLODIN, HEXIL, REXIDIN, FLUDENT-CH 0.2% mouth wash.
13. **Cetrimide:** 0.5–3% solution.
    CETAVLON CONCENTRATE: Cetrimide 20% solution.
    SAVLON LIQUID ANTISEPTIC: Chlorhexidine gluconate 1.5% + Cetrimide 3% solution.
    SAVLON/CETAVLEX CREAM: Chlorhexidine HCl 0.1% + Cetrimide 0.5% cream.
    SAVLON HOSPITAL CONCENTRATE: Chlorhexidine gluconate 7.5% + Cetrimide 15% solution.
14. **Dequalinium chloride:** 0.25–1.0%; DEQUADIN 0.25 mg lozenges.
15. **Ethanol:** 70–90%
16. **Isopropanol:** 70–90%
17. **Formaldehyde:** 4% as diluted FORMALIN (37%)
18. **Glutaraldehyde:** 2%
19. **Boric acid:** 4% solution in warm water, 30% in Boroglycerine paint;
    BOROCIDE 10% oint, BOROSPIRIT 10% ear drops.
20. **Silver nitrate:** 1%
21. **Zinc sulfate:** 1–4%; ZINCO-SULFA 0.1% eye drops, THIOSOL 2.5% lotion, THIOSOL FORTE 4% lotion.
22. **Gentian violet:** 0.5–1.0%
23. **Acriflavine:** 0.1–1%; ACRINOL 0.1% cream.
24. **Nitrofurazone:** 0.2–1.0%; FURACIN 0.2% cream, soluble oint, powder.

ECTOPARASITICIDES

1. **Permethrin:** *For scabies:* PERMITE, HH-MITE, NOMITE 5% cream; apply all over the body except face and head; wash after 8–12 hours; SCABERID 5% cream, 1% soap; SCABPER 5% lotion, ZEROSCAB 5% lotion, 1% soap. *For head lice:* PERLICE, PERMED 1% cream rinse, ELICE 5% lotion; massage about 30 g into the scalp, washoff after 10 min.
2. **Lindane (Gamma hexachlorocyclohexane):**
   For pediculosis: apply to scalp and hair (taking care not to enter eyes), leave for 12–24 hr. (a shower cap may be used for long hair) and then wash off. If lice are still present repeat treatment after 1 week.
   For scabies: the lotion/cream is rubbed over the body (below neck) and a scrub bath taken 12–24 hr later. Single treatment suffices in most patients; can be repeated after a week;
   GAB 1% lotion, ointment; SCABOMA 1% lotion; GAMASCAB 1% lotion, cream; ASCABIOL 1% emulsion with cetrimide 0.1%.
3. **Benzyl benzoate:** Apply 25% emulsion/ointment all over body (except face and neck) after a cleansing bath. Apply 2nd coat next day and wash off 24 hours later;
   DERMIN 25% lotion; SCABINDON 25% oint with DDT 1% and benzocaine 2%,
   BENZYLBENZOATE APPLICATION 25% lotion.
4. **Crotamiton:** Apply 10% lotion/cream twice at 24 hour interval and wash off the next day;
   CROTORAX 10% cream and lotion.
5. **Sulfur:** Apply 10% ointment daily for 3 days followed by soap-water bath on 4th day.
6. **Dicophane (DDT):** Apply 1–2% lotion/ointment all over except face, wash off next day;
   in SCABINDON 1% ointment with benzylbenzoate 25% and benzocaine 2%.
7. **Ivermectin:** 12 mg (0.2 mg/kg) oral single dose for scabies, head and body lice;
   IVERMECTOL, IVERMECT, VERMIN 3, 6 mg tabs, to be taken on empty stomach.

VACCINES

Killed (inactivated) vaccines

Bacterial

- Typhoid - paratyphoid (TAB)
- Vi Typhoid polysaccharide
- Whooping cough (Pertussis)
- Meningococcal
- *Haemophilus influenzae* type B
- Pneumococcal conjugate vaccine (PCV)

Viral

- Poliomyelitis inactivated (IPV; Salk vaccine)
- Fractional-dose inactivated polio vaccine (fIPV)
- Rabies (purified chick embryo cell; PCEV)
- Rabies (Human diploid cell; HDCV)
- Rabies (Vero cell; PVRV)
- Influenza
- Hepatitis B
- Hepatitis A
- Japnese encephalitis (inactivated)

Live attenuated vaccines

Bacterial

- Bacillus Calmette-Guerin (BCG)
- Typhoid Ty 21a (oral)

Viral

- Poliomyelitis oral vaccine (OPV, Sabin)
- Mumps (Live atte.)
- Measles (Live atte.)
- Rubella (Live atte.)
- Varicella (Live atte.)
- Rotavirus (Live atte.)
- Japanese encephalitis (Live atte.)

Toxoids

- Tetanus (fluid/adsorbed)
- Diphtheria (adsorbed)

Combined vaccines

Double antigen: Diphtheria toxoid + tetanus toxoid (DT-DA)
Triple antigen: Diphtheria toxoid + tetanus toxoid + pertussis vaccine (DPT)
Pentavalent vaccine: DPT + Hepatitis B + H. *influenzae* type B vaccines
Measles + mumps + rubella vaccine (MMR)

Preparations

1. **Typhoid, Paratyphoid A, B (TAB vaccine):** 0.5 ml s.c. 2–3 injections at 2–4 week intervals.
2. **Vi Typhoid polysaccharide vaccine:** 0.5 ml s.c./i.m. once, may be repeated after 3 years;
3. **Typhoid: Ty 21a oral vaccine:** 3 caps taken in 3 doses on alternate days in-between meals; TYPHORAL *S. typhi* strain Ty21A 10^9 organism per cap.
4. **Whooping cough (pertussis) vaccine:** 0.25–0.5 ml s.c./i.m. 3 doses at 4 week intervals in infants and children below 5 years age.
5. **Meningococcal A & C vaccine:** 0.5 ml s.c./i.m. single dose; MENINGOCOCCAL A & C, MENCEVAX A & C 0.5 ml amp, 5 ml vial.
6. **Pneumococcal conjugate vaccine:** 0.5 ml i.m. PREVNAR-13, PNEUMOVAX-23 0.5 ml single dose vial.
7. **Haemophilus influenzae type B (Hib) vaccine:** 0.5 ml i.m. 3 doses at 8 weeks gap for infants 2–6 months, ACT-HIB 0.5 ml inj. 2 doses for those 7–11 months age; only 1 dose for those >1 year; HIB-TITER 0.5 ml and 5.0 ml vial.

8. **Bacillus Calmette-Guérin (BCG) vaccine:** 0.05 ml (neonate) 0.1 ml (older infants and children) intracutaneous injection in deltoid region.
9. **Oral poliovirus vaccine (OPV, Sabin vaccine):** 0.5 ml dropped directly in the mouth at birth and at 6, 10, 14 weeks, booster dose at 15–18 month and at school entry.
10. **Inactivated poliomyelitis vaccine (IPV, Salk vaccine):** 0.5 ml i.m. 3 injections at 4–6 week intervals and then 6–12 months later, booster doses every 5 years.

    Fractional dose inactivated polio vaccination (fIPV): 0.1 ml of IPV injected intradermally (i.d.) at 6 and 14 weeks of age.
11. **Purified chick embryo cell vaccine (PCEV):** 2.5 IU/ml inj; 0.1 ml intradermal (i.d.) over deltoid of both arms on days 0, 3, 7 and over one arm only on days 28 and 90 (total 8 injections) for post exposure prophylaxis of rabies; for primary prophylaxis 3 doses of 0.1 ml i.d. on days 0, 7 and 28; RABIPUR 1 ml inj.
12. **Human diploid cell vaccine (HDCV):** 2.5 i.u./ml inj; 0.2 ml i.d. over both deltoids on days 0, 3 and 7 and over one only on days 28 and 90 (total 8 injections), for post exposure prophylaxis of rabies; for primary prophylaxis 3 doses of 0.1 ml each i.d. on days 0, 7 and 28; MIRV-HDC 2.5 IU inj.
13. **Purified vero cell rabies vaccine (PVRV):** 2.5 i.u./ml inj; 0.2 ml i.d. over both deltoids on days 0, 3 and 7 and over one only on days 28 and 90 (total 8 injections) for post exposure prophylaxis of rabies; for primary prophylaxis 3 doses of 0.1 ml each i.d. on days 0, 7 and 28; VERORAB 1 ml inj; VEROVAX-R 0.5 ml inj.
14. **Influenza virus vaccine:** 0.25 ml (6 month–3 year age), 0.5 ml (> 3 year age) i.m. 2 injections 1–2 months apart; VAXIGRIP 0.5 ml prefilled syringe; FLUARIX 0.5 ml single dose pre filled syringe.
15. **Hepatitis B vaccine:** 1 ml i.m. in deltoid muscle at 0, 1, 6 months (children < 10 yr 0.5 ml injection in the thigh); ENGERIX-B, ENIVAC-HB 1 ml (single dose) and 10 ml (multiple dose) vials.
16. **Hepatitis A vaccine:** 0.5 ml i.m. single dose, may be repeated after 6 months; AVAXIM 0.5 ml prefilled syringe, HAVRIX 0.5 ml inj.

17. **Measles vaccine live attenuated:** 1000 $TCID_{50}$ s.c. single dose; ROUVAX, RIMEVAX, M-VAC 1000 $TCID_{50}$/vial inj.
18. **Rubella vaccine:** 1000 $TCID_{50}$ i.m./s.c. single dose; R-VAC 1000 $TCID_{50}$ in 0.5 ml inj.
19. **Measles-Mumps-Rubella (MMR) vaccine:** 0.5 ml i.m./deep s.c. single dose; TRIMOVAX lyophilized measles 1000 $TCID_{50}$ of Schwarz strain, mumps 5000 $TCID_{50}$ and rubella 1000 $TCID_{50}$ per unit dose (0.5 ml) vial. TRESIVAC lyophilized measles 5000 $TCID_{50}$ of Edmonston Zagreb strain, mumps 5000 $TCID_{50}$ and rubella 4000 $TCID_{50}$ per unit dose (0.5 ml) vial.
20. **Varicella vaccine:** 0.5 ml s.c. single dose for children 1–12 years, and 2 doses 6–10 weeks apart in those >12 years. VARILRIX, OKAVAX 0.5 ml inj.
21. **Rotavirus vaccine (RVV):** 0.5 ml (5 drops) orally to infants at 6, 10 and 14 weeks age; ROTAVAC 0.5 ml single dose vial.
22. **Japanese encephalitis vaccines:**
    Live attenuated SA14-14-2 JE vaccine 0.5 ml s.c. × 2 doses; (JEVAX, JEEV)
    Inactivated JE vaccine (Kolar 821564 xy strain; (JENVAC)
23. **Tetanus toxoid:** 0.5 ml i.m. (also s.c.) 2 doses 4–6 weeks apart for primary immunization, booster dose every 10 years, or after a risky wound; TETANUS TOXOID ADSORBED 0.5 ml amp, 5.0 ml vial.
24. **Diphtheria toxoid:** 0.5 ml i.m. 2–3 injections 4–6 weeks apart in children below 6 years, booster doses after 1 year and at school entry.
25. **Double antigen (Diphtheria-Tetanus toxoids):** 0.5 ml i.m. 2–3 injections 4–8 weeks apart; DUAL ANTIGEN 0.5 ml amp, 5 ml vial.
26. **Triple antigen (Diphtheria-Pertussis-Tetanus, DPT):** 0.5 ml i.m. 2–3 injections 4–8 weeks apart between 3–9 months age, booster dose at 18 months age; TRIPVAC 0.5 ml amp, 10 ml multidose vial.
27. **Pentavalent vaccine:** (Triple antigen + Hepatitis B vaccine + *H. influenzae* type b vaccine) 0.5 ml i.m. to infants at 6, 10 and 14 weeks age.

ANTISERA AND IMMUNOGLOBULINS

Antisera (from Horse)
Tetanus antitoxin (ATS)
Gas gangrene antitoxin (AGS)
Diphtheria antitoxin (ADS)
Antirabies serum (ARS)
Antisnake venom polyvalent (ASV)

Immunoglobulins (Human)
Normal human gamma globulin
Anti-D immunoglobulin
Tetanus immunoglobulin
Rabies immunoglobulin
Hepatitis-B immunoglobulin

Preparations

1. Tetanus antitoxin (ATS): Prophylactic 1500–3000 IU, i.m. or s.c.; therapeutic 50,000–100,000 IU part i.v. and rest i.m.;
   TETANUS ANTITOXIN 750 IU, 1500 IU, 5000 IU, 10,000 IU, 20,000 IU, and 50,000 IU in 1–10 ml ampoules.
   ANTI-TET 10,000 IU inj.
2. Gasgangrene antitoxin (AGS): Prophylactic 10,000 IU; therapeutic 30,000–75,000 IU s.c./i.m./i.v.;
   AGGS 10,000 IU amp.
3. Diphtheria antitoxin (ADS): 20,000–40,000 IU i.m. or i.v. for pharyngeal/laryngeal disease of upto 48 hour duration. Higher dose (upto 100,000 IU may be needed).
   DIPHTHERIA ANTITOXIN 10,000 IU in 10 ml amp.
4. Antirabies serum (ARS): Upto 40 IU/kg infiltrated round the bite wound; IMORAB 1000 IU/5 ml inj.
5. Antisnake venom polyvalent: 20 ml i.v. (1 ml/min) repeated 1–6 hourly till symptoms of envenomation disappear (total upto 300 ml); ANTISNAKE VENOM SERUM POLYVALENT, ASVS lyophilized vial to be reconstituted with 10 ml distilled water; each ml of reconstituted serum neutralizes 0.6 mg cobra, 0.6 mg Russel's viper, 0.45 mg of saw scaled viper and 0.45 mg of Krait venoms.

6. **Normal human gamma globulin:** 0.02–0.1 ml/kg i.m.; GAMMALIN, GLOBUNAL, Sii GAMMA GLOBULIN, GAMAFINE 10%, 16.5% injection in 1, 2 ml amps; For i.v. use; sii IVGG 0.1–0.4 g/kg/day; 0.5, 1.0, 2.5 g vials, IMMUNOREL 10 g/100 ml inj.
7. **Rho(D) immune globulin:** (*See* p. 198)
8. **Tetanus immunoglobulin:** Prophylactic 250–500 IU, therapeutic 3000–6000 IU i.m. and/or 250–500 IU intrathecal inj.: TETAGLOBULINE, TETAGAM 250 IU/ml inj.
9. **Rabies immunoglobulin (HRIG):** 20 IU/kg infiltrated round the bite on the day of exposure, BERIRAB-P 300 IU/2 ml and 750 IU/5 ml inj; RABGLOB 300 IU/2 ml inj.
10. **Hepatitis B immunoglobulin:** 1000–2000 IU (adults), 32–48 IU/kg (children) to be administered within 7 days of exposure; HEPAGLOB 100 IU (0.5 ml) 200 IU (1 ml) per vial for i.m. inj.

Index of Nonproprietary Names of Drugs

A

B

D

E

H

I

J

K

L

M

P

Q

R

T

U

V

W

Index of Proprietary (Brand) Names of Drugs

A

B

C

D

E

F

G

H

I

M

O

P

S

T

U

V